HEP Guide to Long Island
FarmStands

HEP Guide to Long Island
FarmStands
Farmers Markets, CSA, and Local Purveyors

Edited by Charles Monaco
with contributions by
Brian Halweil and Geraldine Pluenneke

photos and paintings by Robbi Goldberg

New York | Sag Harbor
Harbor Electronic Publishing
www.HEPDigital.com
2006

Copyright 2006 Harbor Electronic Publishing
Library of Congress Control Number: 2006930084
ISBN 13: 978-1-932916-26-3 (paper)
ISBN 10: 1-932916-26-1 (paper)
ISBN 13: 978-1-932916-27-0 (eBook)
ISBN 10: 1-932916-27-X (eBook)

Printed in the United States of America.
First printing: July 2006

Contributions by Brian Halweil and Geraldine Pluenneke ©
2006 and earlier in the names of the authors. (Versions of
some of the articles have previously appeared elsewhere.)

Photos and Paintings by Robbi Goldberg © 2006 and earlier
in the name of the artist.

Cover design by Joseph Dunn

A NOTE ON THE TYPE
The body font is Hoefler Text, designed by Jonathan Hoefler
in 1991 for Apple to demonstrate the variety and flexibility of
digital typesetting. It evokes the classic faces Garamond and
Caslon. The articles are set in Gill Sans.

Guide to Long Island FarmStands

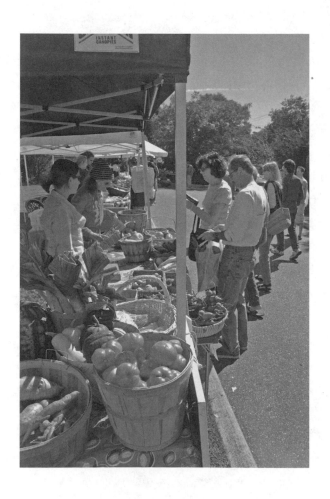

Introduction

Welcome to the first edition of the *HEP Guide to Long Island Farm-Stands, Farmers Markets, CSA, and Local Purveyors*!

Our aim has been to put in your hands an effective and comprehensive guide to the local farm scene on Long Island. Our lengthy list includes all of the farmstands in Nassau and Suffolk counties that we could identify. (If your favorite isn't here, let us know. We'll be sure to include them in the next edition. Email *Jim@Peconic.org.*)

We're inspired by the Slow Food movement, which encourages us all to eat local and seasonal. You'll find information about Slow Food, Community Supported Agriculture, and the farmers market movement here, as well.

And we've also included local Long Island food purveyors — fishmongers, bakers, cheese-makers, honey and jam manufacturers, and the like. If it's local, it's good!

Farmstands run the gamut from a small shelf of extras from the garden to industrial sheds with coolers and freezers, Hawaiian pineapples and California oranges. One of our aims is to give you a sense of what you can expect from one stand or another: is all the produce local? is it organic? what is the variety? Let us know what your experiences have been. We'll include them in the next edition.

Note: Within each section the farmstands are listed — roughly — in geographical order from west to east and from north to south.

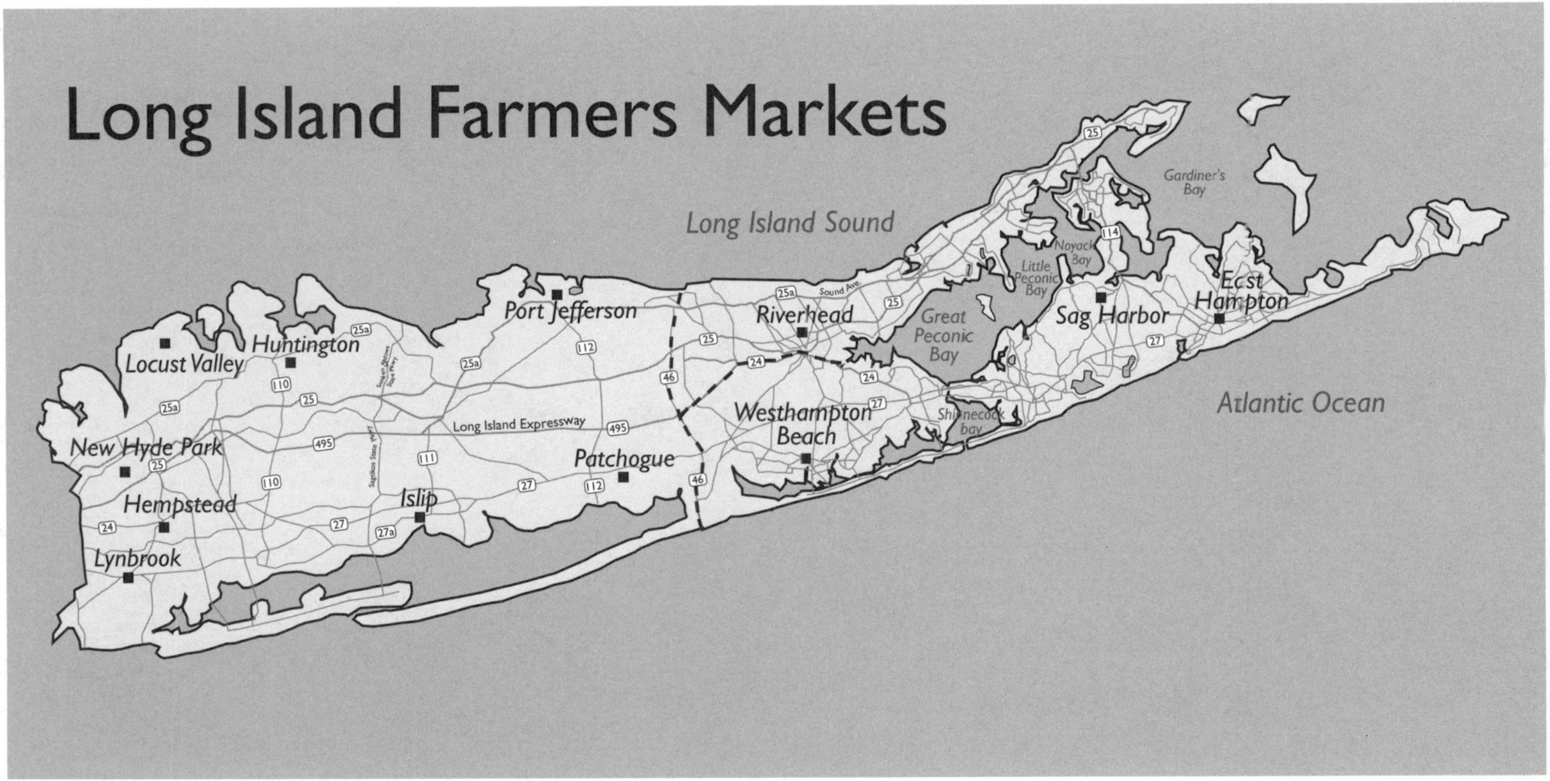

Long Island Farmers Markets
Long Island Sound
Gardiner's Bay
Atlantic Ocean
Locust Valley
Huntington
New Hyde Park
Hempstead
Lynbrook
Islip
Port Jefferson
Patchogue
Long Island Expressway
Riverhead
Sound Ave.
Westhampton Beach
Great Peconic Bay
Little Peconic Bay
Noyack Bay
Shinnecock bay
Sag Harbor
East Hampton

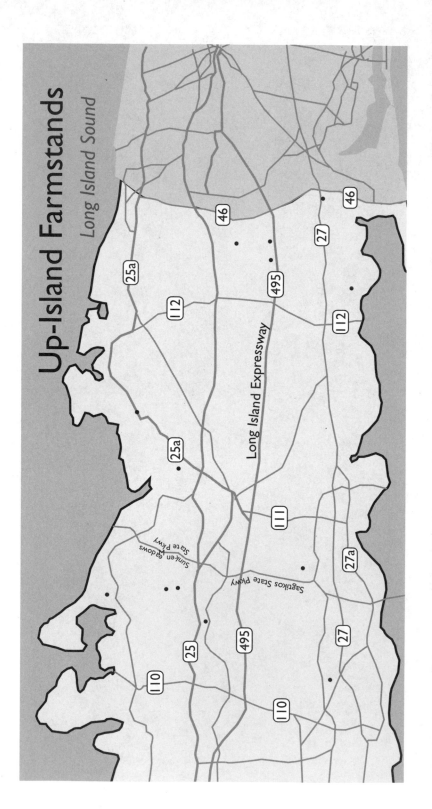

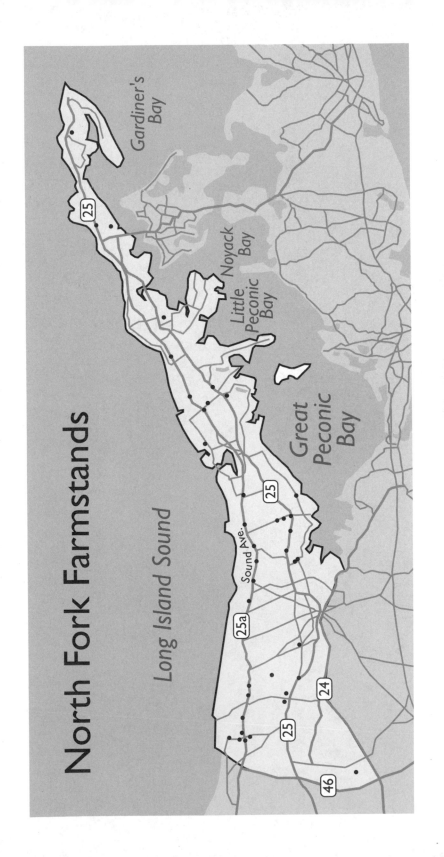

North Fork Farmstands

Long Island Sound

Gardiner's Bay

Noyack Bay

Little Peconic Bay

Great Peconic Bay

Sound Ave.

25

25a

25

24

46

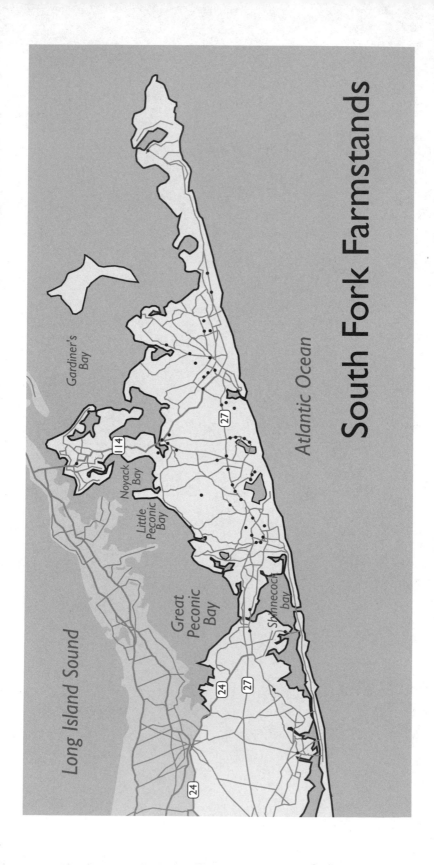

South Fork Farmstands

Long Island Sound

Gardiner's Bay

Atlantic Ocean

Noyack Bay

Little Peconic Bay

Great Peconic Bay

Shinnecock bay

114

27

24

27

24

South Fork FarmStands

Olish's Farmstand

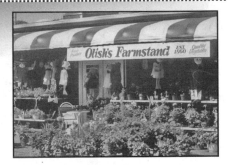

111 Main St.
Eastport, NY 11941
631-325-0539

Dean's

Library Avenue
Westhampton Beach,
NY 11977

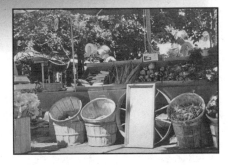

Hampton Fruit and Vegetable

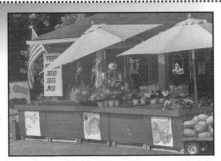

Montauk Highway
East Quogue, NY 11942

Nurel Farms

226 E. Montauk Hwy.
Hampton Bays, NY
11946
631-723-2765

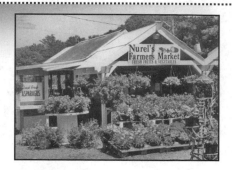

Proprietor: Tony Nurel

Hank's Farmstand

324 County Road 39
Southampton, NY 11968
631-726-4667
hankspumpkintown.com

Proprietors: Hank and Lynne Kraszewski

Directions: 495 East to exit 70; Follow signs for Rte. 27 East (Montauk). Once 4 lanes narrows into two lanes, go through 5 more lights. Located on right.

Season: June to mid-September.

Hours: 7 days a week, 9:30 A.M. to 6 P.M.

Products: Pick your own berries, plus all locally grown fruits and vegetables, jams, baked goods, cut flowers.

Special Events: U-pick strawberries during June. U-pick raspberries and blackberries during July and August.

Hank's Pumpkin-town

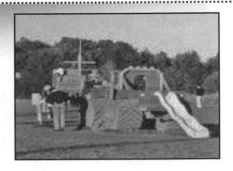

149 Montauk Highway
Water Mill, NY 11976
631-726-4667
hankspumpkintown.com

Proprietors: Hank and Lynne Kraszewski

Directions: 495 East to exit 70; Follow signs for Rte. 27 East (Montauk). Once 4 lanes narrows into two lanes, go through 7 more lights and make a left. Located 1/2 mile on right.

Season: Mid-September to October 31.

Hours: 7 days a week, 9:30 A.M. to 6 P.M.

Products: Huge selection of fall items, pumpkins, gourds, Indian corn, mums, straw bales, baked goods, apples etc.

Special Events: Every weekend: 8-acre interactive corn maze, wagon rides, roasted corn, pony rides. School tours welcome, reservations necessary.

About: Pumpkintown evolved from years of declining potato prices forcing the Kraszewski family to supplement their acreage with other crops. Today the farm consists of over 400 acres located on many different parcels. Potatoes are still grown on the farm as well as strawberries, raspberries, blackberries, sweet corn, field corn, vegetables, flowers and, of course, pumpkins.

Green Thumb of Watermill

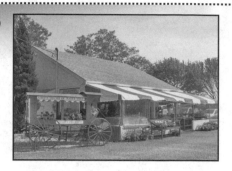

829 Montauk Highway
Water Mill, NY 11976
631-726-1900
fax 631-726-6126

Proprietor: The Raymond Halsey Family

Directions: LIE to exit 70, head south to Sunrise Highway/ Route 27; head east past Water Mill village. Located on right side.

Season: Early May to early December.

Hours: 7 days a week, 9 A.M. to 5 P.M.

Products: Over 300 varieties of certified organic vegetables, herbs, berries, and flowers. Many types of herb and vegetable starter plants for the garden.

Special Events: CSA memberships available in Huntington, Brooklyn, Queens, and Water Mill.

About: CSA. The Green Thumb celebrates its forty-fifth year this summer. The Halsey family has continuously farmed this land since the 1600s.

Halsey Farmstand

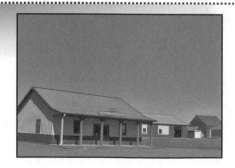

513 Deerfield Road
at Head of Pond Road
Water Mill, NY 11976
halseyfarm@aol.com

Proprietor: Adam Halsey

Directions: Turn north off Montauk Hwy. onto Deerfield Rd. Located one mile north at the intersection of Head of Pond Rd.

Season: July 1 to November 30.

Hours: 7 days a week, 8 A.M. to 6 P.M.

Products: Wide assortment of vegetables and cut flowers, grown on the farm. Potatoes, melons, corn, tomatoes, beans eggplant, peppers, onions, spinach, lettuce, herbs, carrots, cukes, squash and locally grown fruit.

About: A family farm since 1747. All produce picked throughout the day as it is sold.

Amy's Flowers and Mini Milk Pail

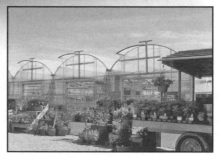

757 Mecox Road
Water Mill, NY 11976
631-537-2565
jennhalsey@milk-pail.com
milk-pail.com

Proprietors: Jennifer Dupree and Amy Halsey

Season: May 1 to Labor Day.

Hours: 7 days a week, 9 A.M. to 5 P.M.

Products: Unique plants and much more.

Special Events: U-pick apples and pumpkins from September to October; Fri., Sat., Sun., and Holidays 10 A.M. to 5:30 P.M. (see website for more information).

About: Amy's Flowers, a division of the Milk Pail, started business in the Spring of 1994. In the past few years several expansions have taken place and an increased variety of plant material is now available.

The Milk Pail

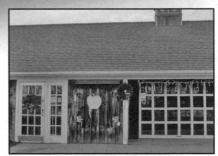

1346 Montauk Highway
Water Mill, NY 11976
631-537-2565
jennhalsey@milk-pail.com
milk-pail.com

Proprietors: Jennifer Dupree and Amy Halsey

Season: Mid-August to mid-April.

Hours: Mon. to Sat., 9:30 A.M. to 5:30 P.M.; Sun., 10 A.M. to 5:30 P.M.

Products: Apples, peaches, pumpkins, pears, blueberries, apple and peach cider, apple and peach pies, apple muffins, apple cider donuts, Vermont cheese, homemade jams, gift packs.

Special Events: Special events.

About: The Milk Pail Country Store began more than 30 years ago. John and Evelyn Halsey, along with their daughters Amy and Jennifer, are the 11th and 12th generation of Halseys carrying on a farming tradition that began more than 350 years ago. Their family farm and orchard is located on the shores of the same Mecox Bay that attracted the first Halsey settlers.

Zaluski Farms

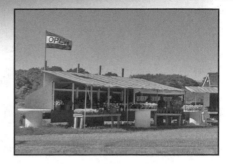

Seven Ponds Road
Water Mill, NY 11976
631-726-6850

Proprietor: Patrick Carroll

Directions: East on Route 39, turn left at the light after the Jitney and proceed to Seven Ponds Road.

Season: May 20 to October 31.

Hours: 7 days a week, 8:30 A.M. to 7 P.M.

Products: Corn, lettuce, tomatoes, peaches, apples, cut flowers, potatoes, sugar-snaps, pumpkins, gourds, hanging baskets, woody ornamentals, and all other local veggies.

About: Zaluski Farm was established in 1907; the farmstand has been in operation since 1985. The farmstand grows what it sells.

Seven Ponds Orchard

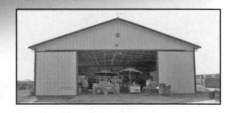

65 Seven Ponds Road
Water Mill, NY 11976
631-726-5140

Proprietor: Tim Kraszewski

Directions: Located just north of County Rd. 39.

Season: June to October.

Hours: 7 days a week, 9 A.M. to 5 P.M.

Products: Pick-your-own berries, apples.

Fairview Farm at Mecox

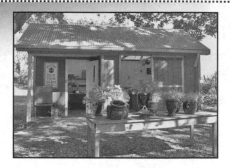

19 Horsemill Lane
Bridgehampton, NY
11932
631-537-1445

Proprietor: Harry Ludlow

Directions: Turn onto Mecox Rd. from Montauk Hwy. between Water Mill and Bridgehampton. At the second stop sign, turn left. We are located at the next intersection, on the corner of Mecox Rd. and Horsemill Lane.

Season: May to October.

Hours: Mon. to Sat., 10 A.M. to 6 P.M. Closed Sun.

Products: Full line of fruits, vegetables, flowers, and herbs. Also Mecox Bay cheeses.

Special Events: A uniquely designed 8 acre corn maze overlooking Mecox Bay and Swan Creek, surrounded by 200 acres of farmland (starting on Labor Day weekend).

Hayground Farmstand

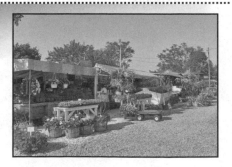

Montauk Highway
Bridgehampton, NY
11932
631-537-1676
fax 631-722-7893

Proprietors: Brad and Lorraine Reeve and sons

Season: April to November.

Hours: 7 days a week, 8 A.M. to 6 P.M.

Products: Asparagus, strawberries, sweet corn, spinach, tomatoes, broccoli cauliflower, brussels sprouts, roasted corn.

Special Events: U-pick strawberries in June.

Babinski Farmstand

291 Lumber Lane
Bridgehampton, NY
11932

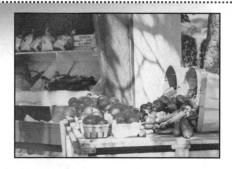

Products: Vegetables, free-range eggs.

Bridgehampton Country Market

2209 Montauk Hwy.
Bridgehampton, NY
11932

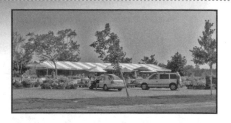

North Sea Farm

1060 Noyac Road
North Sea, NY 11968
631-283-0735

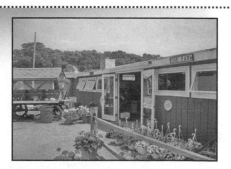

Proprietor: Richie Tate

Directions: Located approx. 4 miles north of Rte. 27.

Season: Year-round.

Products: Chickens, eggs, produce, baked goods.

Tate's Bake Shop

43 North Sea Road
North Sea, NY 11968
631-283-9830
fax 631-283-9844
kathleen@tatesbakeshop.com
tatesbakeshop.com

Proprietor: Kathleen King

Season: Year-round.

Hours: 7 days a week, 6 A.M. to 6 P.M.

Products: All-American scratch baked goods, chocolate-chip cookies, pies, cakes, brownies, and more.

Kilb's Farmstand

Route 114
Shelter Island, NY 11964

Proprietor: Alfred Kilb

Products: Honey, candies, jam.

Card's Farmstand

Shelter Island, NY 11964
631-749-2293

Directions: Located across from Pat & Steve's restaurant.

R & R Farms

12 Cornell Dr. Redwood
Sag Harbor, NY 11963
631-725-3794

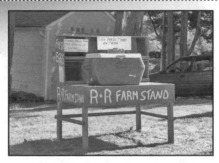

Proprietor: George Speckenbach

Product: Eggs of all sizes.

About: Named for his 12-year-old twin daughters Rachel and Rebecca who get all the double-yolk eggs. George learned dairy in NJ.

The Tomato Lady

291 Main Street
Sag Harbor, NY 11963

Proprietor: Carol Olejnik

Season: August to frost.

Hours: 7 days a week, 10 A.M. to 6 P.M.

Products: Tomatoes, peppers, and more from the Musnicki farm in Bridgehampton.

About: Carol took over from her mother. The farmstand has been in operation for 33 years.

Under the Willow

1726 Bridgehampton Turnpike
Sag Harbor, NY 11963
631-725-5262

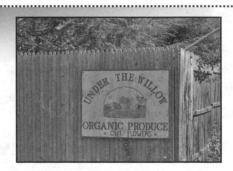

Proprietors: Dale Haubrich and Bette Lacina

Directions: Located just south of Sag Harbor on the east side of Bridgehampton Turnpike.

Season: September to October.

Hours: Fri. and Sat. only, 10 A.M. to 5 P.M.

Products: Organic vegetables of all kinds.

About: Under the Willow was established in 1992 but Dale has been farming organically since 1978. Most of their produce goes to local restaurants and markets, and they sell at the Sag Harbor Farmers Market. Their produce is also available at Schiavoni's market in Sag Harbor.

Pike Farms

Sagg Main Street
Sagaponack, NY 11962

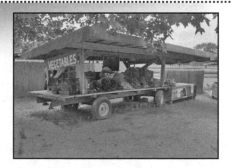

Proprietors: Jim and Jennifer Pike

Directions: Located 1/4 mile south of Rte. 27 on Sagg Main St., Sagaponack (between Bridgehampton and East Hampton).

Season: June to October.

Hours: 7 days a week, 9 A.M. to 7 P.M.

Products: Arugula, tomatoes, zucchini, artichokes, beans, beets, broccoli, brussels sprouts, basil, carrots, cauliflower, sweet corn, cucumbers, eggplant, gourds, leeks, lettuce, onions, peas, peppers, pumpkins, squash, blueberries, strawberries, raspberries, blackberries, peaches, plums, nectarines, cherries, apples, muskmelons, watermelons, bread, cookies, pies, chips, nuts, honey, jams, cut flowers.

Liberty Farm Nursery

651 Main St.
Sagaponack, NY 11962
631-537-8001
fax 631-537-2352

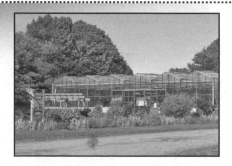

Proprietors: Jeffrey and Kathleen White

Directions: Turn south off Montauk Highway on Sagg Main St. Located two miles down, on the left.

Season: April to October.

Hours: 7 days a week, 9 A.M. to 7 P.M.

Products: Vegetables, herbs, annuals, perennials, cut flowers.

About: A growing part of the White family farm, since 1695.

Marilee Foster

Sagg Main St.
Sagaponack, NY 11962
631-537-1014

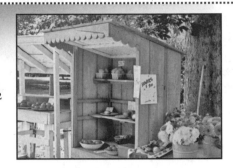

Proprietor: Marilee Foster

Products: A selection of home-grown vegetables including organic potatoes.

Thayer's

345 Sagg Main St.
Sagaponack, NY 11962
631-537-0848

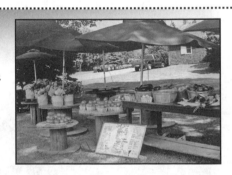

Proprietor: Carrie Crowley

Season: July 4 'til the corn runs out.

Hours: Mon. to Fri., 9 A.M. to 7 P.M.; Fri. and Sat., 9 A.M. to 8 P.M.; Closed Sun.

Products: Flowers, corn, tomatoes, and more.

Lisa and Bill's

Main Street and
Beach Lane
Wainscott, NY 11975

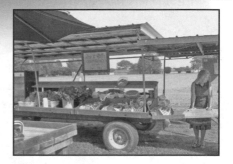

Proprietor: Billy Babinski

Season: June to October 31.

Hours: Seven days, 9 A.M. to 6 P.M.

Products: Strawberries, corn, melons, lettuce, tomatoes, zucchini, peppers, flowers, cookies, pies, and more.

Special Events: U-pick pumpkins in October.

About: The farmstand was established in 1984. The farm dates back 350 years.

Bogo's Food Spa

27 Race Lane
East Hampton, NY 11937
631-00329-1004
fax 631-899-2534
bogo@bogofood.com
bogofood.com

Proprietor: John Bogosian

Directions: From Rte. 27, take a left at the Getty Station onto Toilsome Lane. At the 5-way intersection, go straight. Continue around the sharp curve to the right until you reach the stop sign. Turn to the left, and you are on Race Lane. You will see Hampton's Marketplace on your right. Bogo's Food Spa is located approximately 40 yards on your left hand side.

Season: July to October.

Products: Variety of local produce and other foods. Offers a buying club.

EECO Farm

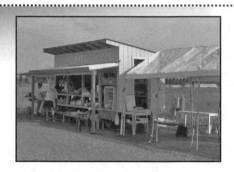

55 Long Lane
East Hampton, NY
11937
631-324-5523
fax 631-329-7590
eecofarm.com

Proprietor: Paul Hamilton, Farm Manager

Directions: Route 114 to Stephen Hands Path. East to Long Lane. South to the farmstand, located on the right across from Iacono's chicken farm.

Season: May to November.

Hours: 7 days a week, 10 A.M. to 6 P.M.

Products: Wide variety of produce.

Special Events: Many seminars and special events. See the website for schedules.

About: EECO (East End Community Organic) Farm is a grassroots, not-for-profit educational organization growing sustainable agricultural enterprises for the health of the community. EECO operates a community organic farm for the benefit of area residents, in collaboration with the Town of East Hampton, which owns a 42-acre parcel of prime agricultural land across from East Hampton High School. The community farm is an outdoor classroom for learning about sustainable agricultural practices, organic yard and lawn care and how to preserve our natural resources. In addition to the farm, EECO provides acreage for 120 community gardens where members grow their own vegetables.

Bistrian Farmstand

Cedar St. at North Main St.
East Hampton, NY 11937
631-324-5936

Proprietors: Sharon and Michael Bistrian

Season: July to September.

Products: Corn.

About: For a long time the Bistrians have sold their corn at a temporary farmstand across from the East Hampton Fire Department.

Iacono Farm

106 Long Lane
East Hampton, NY
11937
631-324-1107

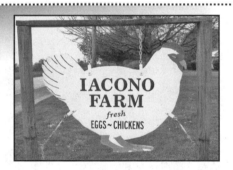

Proprietors: Salvadore and Anthony Iacono

Directions: From Main Street in East Hampton, turn north onto Newtown Lane. Stay on Newtown Lane. Pass the High School onto Long Lane. Located about 1/2 mile down, marked by a sign in the shape of a chicken.

Season: Year-round.

Hours: Mon. and Wed. to Sat., 9:30 A.M. to 5 P.M. (Closed noon to 1 P.M. for lunch); Sun., 10 A.M. to noon; closed Tue.

Products: Fresh-killed chickens raised on the farm. All free-range and antibiotic and hormone-free. Eggs.

LKL Farmstand

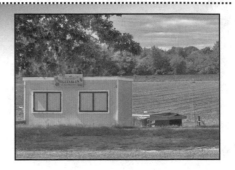

Pantigo Road
East Hampton, NY
11937
631-267-0046
fax 631-267-2269

Proprietor: Lynn Bistrian Dale

Directions: On Route 27 between East Hampton and Amagansett. The yellow farmstand on the north side of the road.

Season: July 1 to November 1.

Hours: 7 days a week, 8 A.M. to 7 P.M.

Products: Vegetables, fruit, jams and jellies, fresh-baked pies, flowers. Cut your own sunflowers, pick your own pumpkins.

Special Events: Animals to pet (donkey, pony, rabbit).

About: Family owned and run.

Regina's Farmstand

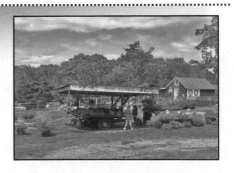

42 Oak View Highway
East Hampton, NY
11937
631-329-3117
fax 631-329-6010

Proprietor: Regina B. Whitney

Directions: From East Hampton take North Main St. one mile. Make a left on Oak View Highway. Located 1/4 mile on right.

Season: Mother's Day to October; Thanksgiving to New Year's.

Hours: Thu. to Mon., 9 A.M. to 7 P.M. Closed Tue. and Wed.

Products: Organic vegetables, cut flowers, potted plants.

Special Events: Floral design for parties and weddings.

Hardscrabble Farmstand

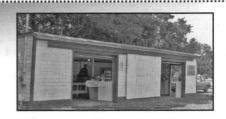

Route 114 at Stephen
Hands Path
East Hampton, NY

Season: July 'til the corn runs out.

Round Swamp Farm

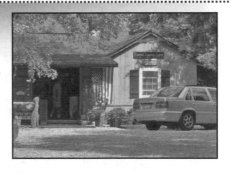

184 Three Mile Harbor
Road
East Hampton, NY
11937
631-324-4438
fax 631-324-3393

Proprietor: Carolyn Snyder

Directions: Montauk Highway east to North Main Street north, bear left onto Three Mile Harbor Road.

Season: April to December.

Hours: Mon. to Sat., 8 A.M. to 6 P.M.; Sun., 8 A.M. to 2 P.M.

Products: Fruits, vegetables, homemade baked goods, prepared foods, and salads; locally caught fish, jams and staples.

About: The Round Swamp farmstand is an interesting mix: part traditional farmstand, part local high end market, with a small fish counter as well. A National Bicentennial Farm, it has been run by the Lester family for over 250 years.

Pig Pen Produce

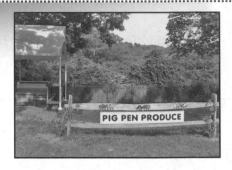

240 Three Mile
Harbor Road
East Hampton, NY
11937

Directions: About three miles north of town.

Amagansett Farmer's Market

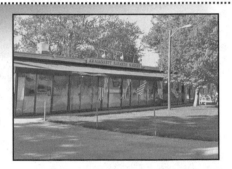

Main St.
Amagansett, NY 11930
631-267-3894

About: More of a general store, but it is seasonal and it does carry some local produce.

Vicki's Veggies

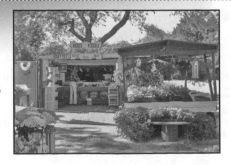

Montauk Highway
Amagansett, NY 11930
631-267-8820

About: If you live in Montauk this is about your closest farm-stand.

Little Farmstand

Spring Close Highway
Amagansett, NY 11930
631-267-6150

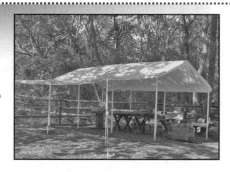

Directions: Near the Spring Close Tree Farm.

Quail Hill Community Farm

Side Hill Lane
 at Deep Lane
Amagansett, NY 11930
631 267 8492

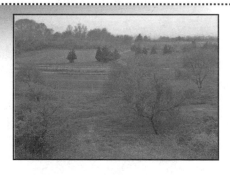

Proprietor: Scott Chaskey for the Peconic Land Trust

Directions: No farmstand.

Season: June to November.

Hours: Sat. and Tue., 8 A.M. to 6 P.M.

Products: More than 200 varieties of vegetables, herbs, fruits, and flowers.

Special Events: CSA. Winter shares also available from November through February: root vegetables, garlic, onions, etc.

About: Located on land that was donated to the Peconic Land Trust by Deborah Ann Light in 1989, Quail Hill Farm serves as an example of the Trust's commitment to actively care for the land it protects. The farm comprises 25 acres serving 200 families. Farm members purchase a share each year which enables them to harvest fresh vegetables, fruits, and flowers throughout the growing season. Quail Hill Farm is certified organic by, and is a member of NOFA-NY (Northeast Organic Farming Association) and is a member of the biodynamic Farming and Gardening Association. The Farm is an innovative model of community-supported agriculture and provides the public with an opportunity to participate in the stewardship of protected land.

Balsam Farms

Town Lane at
Windmill Lane
Amagansett, NY 11930
631-255-9417
balsamfarms.com

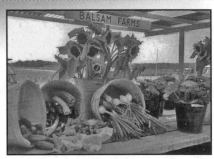

Proprietor: Alexander Balsam

Directions: Just west of Amagansett, turn north onto Windmill Lane and go all the way to the end.

Season: July to October.

Hours: 7 days a week, variable, usually 9:30 A.M. to 6 P.M.

Products: Sweet corn, new potatoes, fingerlings, tomatoes of all kinds, summer squash, patty pan squash, cukes, edamame, sweet potatoes, raspberries, green and wax beans, onions, shallots, leeks, peppers, eggplant, watermelon, musk melon, basil, cilantro, broccoli, pumpkins, gourds, flowers.

About: Started in 2002 on 10 acres, Balsam Farms, LLC, now farms 43 acres of vegetables. Most of their crops are grown without the use of synthetic chemicals and they do not retail anyone else's produce. They also sell to high quality restaurants, specialty food shops and other farmstands throughout the Hamptons.

The Sagg Strip

Pike Farms
Sagg Main Street
Sagaponack, NY

Thayer's
345 Sagg Main Street
Sagaponack, NY

Liberty Farms
Sagg Main Street
Sagaponack, NY

Marilee Foster
Sagg Main Street
Sagaponack, NY

The mouthwatering attractions pop up one after another, beckoning drivers like the all-you-can-eat dinner offers in Vegas. Except the temptation is more healthy. And less gaudy.

There's an oversized tomato. A shimmering ear of sweet corn. A hand-painted menu of available victuals.

Sagg Main Street in Sagaponack might hold the greatest density of farmstands on the East End. It's natural to stop here for food, and not just because this thoroughfare historically connected the farms of Sagaponack with the port of Sag Harbor and markets elsewhere. The strip is also conveniently on the way to and from some prime beaches.

While today's stands all offer Long Island standards, from cabbage and corn to turnips and tomatoes, they differ in style and aesthetics. They shrink in size as you head towards the ocean. And they stretch back in time to the earliest notion of stands set up to sell excess from the farm's kitchen garden.

Closest to the highway and just past from Loaves & Fishes, the first stand sits against a pastel backdrop of red, yellow, and purple zinnias. "It's somewhat strategic," Jim Pike said of the planting. "The flowers do make a nice backdrop. People like coming here just for the experience of looking around."

In fact, the craving can generate a small traffic clot here on a busy weekend afternoon. Or even at 9AM on a Tuesday morning in August. "It's tough getting set up sometimes," said Jennifer Pike, often seen behind the stand while her husband drives a tractor in nearby fields.

It still beats selling cauliflower from a truck on Highway 27, her husband added. "It's very unpleasant on the highway," Mr. Pike said, distracted by a diesel Mercedes idling nearby. "There's the constant din of traffic."

Relatively speaking, Pike Farms is deluxe, sprawling with several wooden trailers retrofitted with wooden roofs and filled with corn, melons, tomatoes, and baskets of most produce you'd find at your neighborhood green grocer. It opens towards the end of May — "from strawberry season to Thanksgiving" — and is noteworthy for being one of the first local farmers with homegrown tomatoes, by planted them in April under "poly low tunnels."

But Mr. Pike, who started farming on the East End two decades ago, is also a relative newcomer. Originally from Westchester County, he worked with several area farmers before opening his own stand in 1987. He now rents roughly 65 acres in and around Sagaponack and grows a dizzying selection of vegetables for his stand.

"We grow a lot of our own stuff and people do appreciate that," said Mr. Pike, as he walked past a cart loaded down with half a dozen different tomatoes (from orange and yellow cherries to beefsteaks in shades of red and pink), another cart piled with muskmelon, and baskets packed with beans, berries, and basil, not to mention potatoes and peppers.

Like many East End farmstands, they supplement their own supply in the early summer, occasionally bringing in out-of-season produce to keep the stand full of popular items. They also offer local honey and baked goods. "We try to have a lot of options because lots of people do all their shopping here," said Mrs. Pike.

The next stand down the road, over the railroad bridge and past the Sagg General Store, shaded by multi-colored umbrellas, is run by Carrie Thayer Crowley and Terry Crowley. Set up in front of the house and potato fields where Mrs. Crowley grew up, the stand opens from July 4th "'til the corn's gone and the tomatoes are gone," according to Mr. Crowley.

The couple has been operating the stand seasonally since 1985, making it the oldest on the strip. They do most of the picking and sorting themselves, with occasional help from family and some farmworkers. Neighborhood kids or nieces and nephews often run the stand.

The couple grows their own tomatoes and corn on several acres, but bring in much of the other produce and fruit from elsewhere. They offer pies, cakes, and breads baked nearby.

And it's the only Sagg stand that offers eggs, a limited and colorful supply grown by Carrie's brother that usually sells out early each day. "People fight for them," said Mrs. Crowley.

But the stand is best known for its flowers. "We can't keep them cut," said Mrs. Crowley. "The snapdragons are big sellers." Mr. Thayer adds: "People like how Carrie arranges them."

Mrs. Crowley remembered two other seasonal stands on the street from her childhood: one set up by Ms. Albright and another by the Babinskis. These stands didn't coincide with the newer ones, so the road never supported more than three.

"It's a busy stretch, so I think we're fortunate for that," she added. "Lots of people like to do business on the backroads." On summer afternoons, cars loaded with surfboards and beach chairs pile up, and sunbathers help empty the stand.

Even closer to the Atlantic coast, kitty-corner to Liberty Farm Nursery, the greenhouse that sells flowers, herbs, and other potted plants, a sign declares "Vegetables" in a stenciled, black font.

"I just refer to it as 'the stand'," said Marilee Foster, who has been selling roadside for seven years. The blue-gray structure, smaller than most city closets, holds Ms. Foster's wares, displayed in colorful home-turned bowls and other pottery and labeled with home-made signs featuring veggie characters. When her harvest swells in late summer, she adds a table she built herself and a wire garden stand salvaged from the yard. "Everything down there has a hue of blue," she said. "I'm overtly interested in how it looks."

The strictly self-serve stand, is the first on Sagg Main to set out produce each year, offering asparagus and lettuce in early May. It's also the only stand that exclusively sells homegrown crops, and so shoppers can use it to track the state of the local harvest.

Recent visitors could find organic potatoes, eggplant, zucchini, and some unusual looking tomatoes that suffered in the heavy rains earlier this month. "The heirlooms look really rather terrible," she said. The taste hasn't suffered at all, and so Ms. Foster has been packing boxes of cracked fruit to sell for sauce.

"No one in the family had an actual garden," she remembered, explaining the genesis of the stand seven years ago. "We were growing all the potatoes in the world and had to go somewhere else for groceries. That was strange."

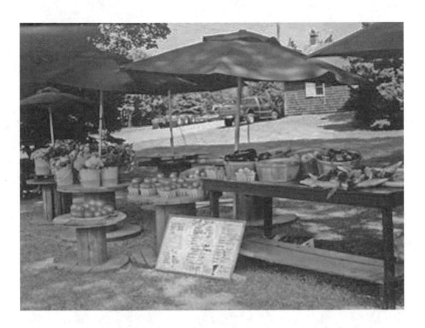

The handful of family and friends that helped to hatch the idea shortly moved onto other projects, leaving Ms. Foster to mind the kitchen garden and stand. Today, the family has all the vegetables it needs, and plenty left to sell.

"It started as a way to learn about vegetable farming," she said, "and it's taken on a life of its own."

—*Brian Halweil*

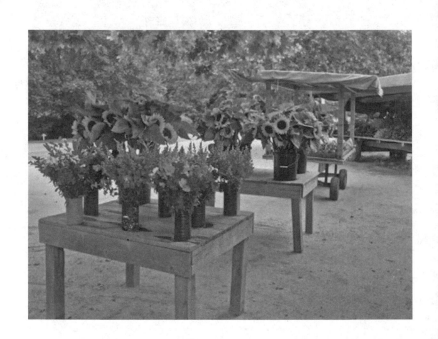

The Zen of Ripeness

The Tomato Lady
291 Main Street
Sag Harbor, NY

Under a canopy of bright beach umbrellas at the southern end of Sag Harbor's Main Street across from Canio's Books, Carol Olejnik sets up shop. Tomato plants create a wall in front of the house: the ersatz privet hedge. A white banner punctuated by three red tomatoes flies above. A no frills sign advertises the wares — pints $3, quarts $6, cherries $3 — and declares "The Tomato Lady's Stand, Est. 1973."

The setting is simple, but the fruit is impeccable.

"I've been doing this for some thirty years," Carol says, as she arranges tomatoes, eggplants, cucumber, and peppers on her fold-out table and shelves. Her mother first started selling tomatoes for some extra money. "My mother and me would pick, and my sister would sell," Carol remembers. "It got so busy in Sag, that now we have to hire a few pickers."

Considering the momentary nodes of congestion at the corner of Glover and Main, everyone is thrilled that Carol is open for business. Carol will be the first to tell you that she's a little late this year, delayed about two weeks by the damp, cold spring that kept tomato growers from getting the plants in the ground.

But if there's anything that Carol knows with certainty, she tells me, it's that the local tomato crop always comes in August. "Anyone selling tomatoes in July is bringing them from somewhere else."

Some of Carol's customers might have left the gates prematurely, but they are now here in hoards. Some swear that these are the best tomatoes in the world, and such accolades have a way of creating their own publicity. One customer visited after attending a party where guests couldn't tear themselves away from the tomato appetizers. "We were in heaven," she remembered.

Carol doesn't doubt it. Something to do with the hot summer days and salty air, she suspects. And something to do with the rich Bridgehampton soil under the Musnicki farm where the crop is raised. "Sag Harbor soil is horrible, but Sagaponack and Bridge have great soil," Carol explains. "That's why they grew the crops and Sag was the port of commerce" — a centuries-old tradition that Carol continues to this day.

An enthusiastic woman asks what the difference is between the yellow and red cherries. "How can I tell you?," Carol says with the emphasis on the "I." "You have to taste it to find out." A bit scared and apologetic, the woman doesn't move. "Go ahead. I'm serious. Taste it. But just one taste per customer," Carol warns.

"There's a guy who comes in every week," Carol says. "He tastes everything and never buys anything."

In lulls between customers, Carol grades the fruit by ripeness. It's a subtle calculus based on palpation and when the fruit will be consumed. "You want for lunch? For dinner? For tomorrow? For the next day?," she asks. "You want some ripies?" This personal attention sets the Tomato Lady's Stand apart from pick-your-own farmstands, and permits a fine-tuning of ripeness that generally evades the fragile nightshade.

"I just sold to a lady who was taking the tomatoes to the city," Carol says. "If they're going to travel in a car, you shouldn't have ripe tomatoes." Carol's tomatoes have been shipped to Vermont, Florida, and even Hawaii. Other folks have taken them down to the Caribbean.

The best way to ripen a tomato, she says, is in a brown, paper bag. "And if you stick a apple or banana in the bag, it speeds the process," she adds.

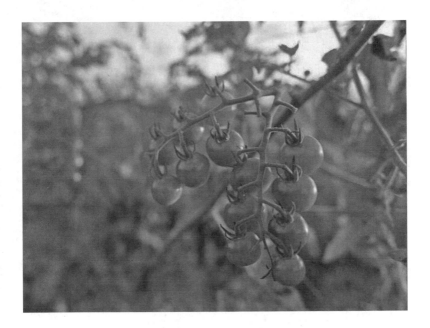

Never keep tomatoes in the sun, Carol continues, and never put them in the refrigerator. "Some people like cool tomatoes, but it changes their flavor," she counters.

"Some city people think that tomatoes should be red, but hard as a rock," Carol laments. "That's what they're used to." Holding a weepy, ripe Beefsteak in her palm, Carol says it should give a little, but she would never pinch it.

In the span of one hour, at least two joyous customers independently compare Carol's yellow cherry tomatoes to "eating candy." Carol doesn't want to publicize the name of this variety, only available here and at the Musnicki stand on Ocean Road.

Some other important advice on cherry tomatoes: "You've got to pop the entire thing in your mouth or else you'll be cleaning tomatoes juice off your clothes."

The stand is filling now with the lunchtime rush. Carol is juggling five customers — two buying for dinner, and three looking for lunch — and she knows three personally.

One young woman is short on cash. "Your credit is good here," Carol says. "You don't have to pay me now. How you gonna get coffee?" The woman says Carol used to be her gym teacher, and Carol rolls her eyes.

"Most of these people grew up coming here," Carol says with visible pride. "Now they're bringing their kids."

Would she call herself an institution, maybe a tradition? "Sometimes it seems like it," she chuckles.

—*Brian Halweil*

Full Moon Organic Suppers

East End Community Organic Farm (EECO)
55 Long Lane
East Hampton, NY

When you mend a broken connection, energy can surge forward. It's happening at the East End Community Organic Farm (EECO), where people schooled in February asparagus and October strawberries are reconnecting with the land and its seasons. You sense the energy when you step onto EECO's 42 acres on Long Lane, less than five minutes from the center of East Hampton.

You find it at the Blue Moon Ball, a sell-out, $150-a head, EECO fund-raiser and auction for 300, at the home of Vicki and Stuart Match Suna. During the auction someone would claim a winning bid to spend a day in the kitchen at Chez Panisse kitchen in Berkeley, CA, and a coveted by-invitation-only dinner at the kitchen's table. But the morning after the farm's first major fundraiser, energy levels would rise even higher as several dozen inner city children from the Boys and Girls Harbor harvested produce at the farm. Early Monday, they gathered in the kitchen of Nick and Toni's and prepared lunch with their EECO bounty under the supervision of the restaurant's chefs.

Every full moon from May until late autumn, a pot luck supper draws scores of the three-year-old farm's member-gardeners and supporting members. There are 104 garden plots – each 20 by 20 feet – that gardeners rent for $75 a year, a bargain Hampton's rental. Three hundred more people hold supporting memberships which entitle them to attend the monthly potlucks. On some Friday evenings, you can catch one couple and their guests seated on cushioned-wicker couches in the center of their plot enjoying cocktails.

At pot lucks you may see Beth Collins, new executive chef of the Ross School, watering seedlings, while her predecessor, Ann Cooper, past president of Women Chefs and Restaurateurs watches her, sipping a glass of wine. In a center green surrounded by gardens, a table full of wine bottles is uncorked. Across the lawn, ribs, paella, salads, and endless dishes are laid on tables. Scratch a community gardener and you'll find an accomplished cook. Artist Lauren Jarrett, EECO co-executive director, tends chicken and sausages on an long steel grill.

Working with plants and watching food grow becomes an elemental experience at EECO, for many a new one. "We have these ex-Merrill-Lynch types who've never planted a thing in their lives. They're here from dawn to dusk," says Kate Plumb, EECO marketing manager. "There's something very grounding about literally being on the ground, working with the ground," says Annie Bliss, the other half of the co-executive directorship. Adds Plumb, "Some of the mishegoss goes away, the craziness, the internal tensions. It's healing."

In addition to the community garden plots, EECO's staff grows almost seven acres of organic row crops, which it sells at its Long Lane farmstand and to over a dozen local restaurants and shops. The farm is leased from the Town of East Hampton. EECO in turn sub-leases one-acre plots to three local commercial farmers. An educational, not-for-profit 501(C)(3) corporation, EECO's aim is to educate the community, particularly children, on the value of sustainable, local, organic agriculture. In the spring, 125 fifth graders and some pre-schoolers surged over the farm, some planting seeds to return in wonder to see robust plants. Plans are underway with East Hampton schools' contracted food service, to put organic EECO foods into the school lunch programs.

EECO soon plans to offer supporting members as well as member-gardeners the chance to pick-your-own produce from its commercial row crops at reduced prices. There will be tiny,

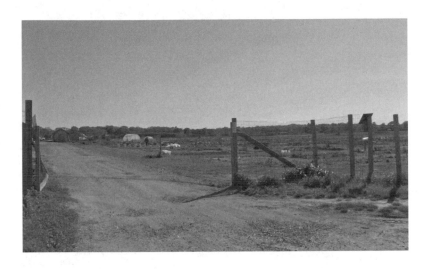

sweet strawberries, peas, beans, flowers, potatoes and pumpkins.

While Christie Brinkley, Peter Cook and Alec Baldwin make the case on one level at the Blue Moon Ball for the wisdom of supporting local foods, EECO is making it on another by feeding some of Long Island's hungry. For each of the last two years, EECO has donated over 2 1/2 tons, or almost 6,000 pounds, of produce, which was distributed through Island Harvest. They also served as a conduit to the hungry for an exceptional, unsung contribution. Last fall, Wainscott farmer Peter Dankowski donated 15,000 pounds of potatoes through EECO and Island Harvest for the hungry. The energy is contagious.

—*Geraldine Pluenneke*

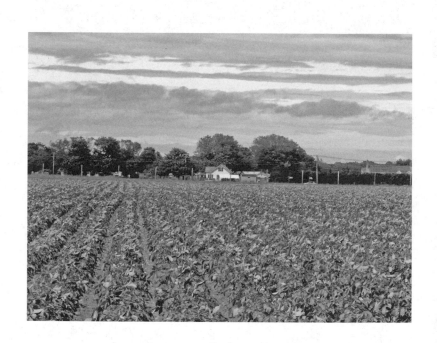

South Fork Purveyors

Paumanok Preserves

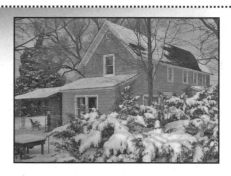

POB 632
Center Moriches, NY
11934
631-878-0619
fax 631-878-6010
paumanokpreserves.com

Proprietor: Joan Bernstcin

Products: Jams, jellies, fruit butters, conserves, compotes, sauces, marmalades and chutneys.

About: Paumanok Preserves are created by Joan Bernstein, a native Long Islander whose family has farmed here for 100 years. The main ingredients are almost all grown regionally. Local fruit in season is picked as available for "farm-to-kitchen freshness."

Jurgielewicz Duck Farm

Barnes Road
Moriches, NY 11955
631-878-2000
fax 631-878-4281

Proprietor: Benjamin Jurgielewicz

Directions: Year-round.

Hours: Mon. to Fri., 8 A.M. to 5 P.M.

Products: Peking ducks.

About: In the business for four generations, one of the last remaining duck farms on Long Island. Although mainly wholesale they do sell by the case (six ducks) direct.

Brewster's Seafood Market

252 East Montauk Highway
Hampton Bays, NY 11946
631-728-3474

Products: Local catches.

Cor-J Seafood

36 Lighthouse Road
Hampton Bays, NY 11946
631-728-5186

Products: Local catches.

The Clam Man

235a North Sea Road
Southampton, NY 11968
631-283-6437
fax 631-283-8102
clamman@clamman.com
clamman.com

Directions: Located south off Montauk Hwy. at North Sea Rd.

Season: Year-round.

Products: Fish, seafood.

Special Events: Catering.

Southampton Publick House

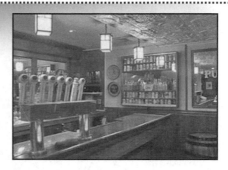

40 Bowden Square
Southampton, NY
11968
631-283-2800
sph@publick.com
publick.com

Proprietor: Phil Markowski, Brewmaster

Directions: Route 27 east into Southampton. Right at the corner of North Sea Road. (7-11 and Gulf Station on the corner). Proceed down North Sea Road. to the second traffic light. Located on the far left hand corner.

Season: Year-round.

Products: Award-winning microbrewery beers and ales, year-round and seasonal.

About: Established in 1996, the Southampton Publick House sells its products to over 40 specialty beer bars and restaurants throughout Long Island and New York City. Since 1998, SPH has been recognized for their brewing excellence at The Great American Beer Festival, Real Ale Festival, and the World Beer Cup.

Blue Duck Bakery

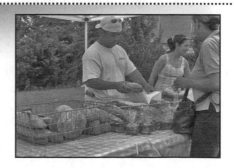

Hampton Road
Southampton, NY
11968
631-204-1701
blueduckbakery@aol.com

Proprietor: Keith

Season: Year-round.

Products: Breads and other baked goods.

Mecox Bay Dairy

Mecox Road
Water Mill, NY 11976
631-537-0335

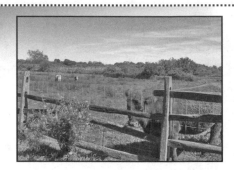

Proprietor: Arthur Ludlow

Products: Award-winning farmstead artisanal cheeses sold at local markets, Sag Harbor and Westhampton Beach Farmers Markets, and at Fairview Farmstand next to the dairy.

Hamptons Honey Company

153 Little Noyac Path
Water Mill, NY 11976
631-537-9495
hamptonshoney.com
frederic@hamptonshoney.com

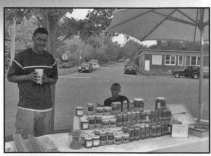

Proprietor: Frederic Rambaud

Directions: Sold locally at most food shops and farmstands and at the Sag Harbor Farmers Market.

Season: May to November.

Products: Honey, jams, syrup.

About: Successor to Don Sausser Apiaries. Long Island's largest apiary, with hives nestled throughout the East End's pristine landscape. The company uses organic bee fields wherever possible and follows strict biodynamic beekeeping principles that avoid the use of plastic hives, antibiotics, and other practices that weaken the bees and compromise the quality of the honey.

Bob's Fish Market
87 North Ferry Road (Rte. 114)
Shelter Island, NY 11964

Products: Local catches.

Le Poème
POB 1566
Shelter Island, NY 11964
631-749-5045

Proprietor: Martine Abitbol

Directions: Sold at the Sag Harbor Farmers Market.

Products: A variety of French bakery goodies.

Special Events: Catering: Mediterranean and Provençal.

Open Minded Organics Mushrooms

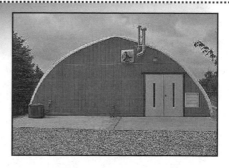

Sag Harbor, NY 11963
631-574-8889
openmindedorganics.com

Proprietor: David Falkowski

Hours: Sold at the Sag Harbor Farmers Market every Sat. during the season.

Products: King Oyster Mushrooms and other varieties of organically grown mushrooms including Shiitaki, Blewitt, Chanterelle, Chicken of the Woods, Hedgehog, Lions Mane (Pom Pom Blanc), Maitake (Hen of the Woods), Morel, Wine Cap Stropharia and others.

About: Open Minded Organics is a family owned and operated company established in 2003. They grow organic mushrooms, and are advocates and supporters of local sustainable agriculture. Each batch of mushrooms is literally hand crafted.

Joe Zaykowski Honey

Sagg Road
Sag Harbor, NY 11963
631-725-1679

Proprietor: Joe Zaykowski

Products: Zaykowski's honey is available at Cromer's, Schiavoni's, the Cheese Shop, Second Nature, Provisions and at local farmstands during the summer months.

Cavaniola's Cheese Shop

89 Division St.
Sag Harbor, NY 11963
631-725-0095
fax 631-725-0504
cavaniolasgourmet@yahoo.com

Products: Local cheeses, artisanal cheeses from around the world, vegetables from the garden, and many other items.

Java Nation

78 Main Street
Sag Harbor, NY 11963
631-725-0500

Products: A variety of coffees and teas. The coffee is fresh-ground on the premises.

Tiger Spud Potato Chips

Sagaponack, NY 11962
631-537-1014

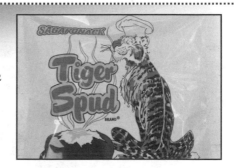

Proprietor: Marilee Foster

The Seafood Shop

Montauk Highway
Wainscott, NY 11975
631-537-0633
mail@theseafoodshop.com
theseafoodshop.com

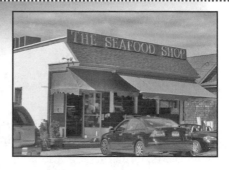

Proprietor: Colin Mather

Directions: Located on Montauk Highway, at the new traffic light in Wainscott.

Season: Year-round.

Hours: 7 days a week, 8 A.M. to 6 P.M.; Fri. and Sat. in summer, 8 A.M. to 8 P.M.

Products: Fish, seafood.

Special Events: Catering, take-out.

About: Evolving from a small summer fish market opened in 1972 by two teachers from local schools, The Seafood Shop is today known by chefs from the Hamptons to New York City for the freshness and selection of their fish. After spending 13 years working at The Seafood Shop under the original owner John Haessler, Colin Mather took over in 2000.

Breadzilla

84 Wainscott-North-
west Road
Wainscott, NY 11975
631-537-0955
breadzilla@aol.com

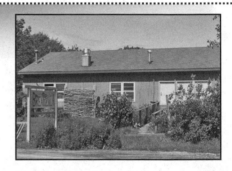

Directions: Located just north of Rte. 27 at the light in Wainscott.

Hours: Tue. to Sat., 8 A.M. to 4 P.M.; Sun., 8 A.M. to 3 P.M.; Closed Mon.

Products: A variety of breads including sourdough, assorted freshly baked breakfast pastries and breads, their own pies, cakes, cookies, tarts, homemade granola, other snack items.

Stuart's Seafood Market

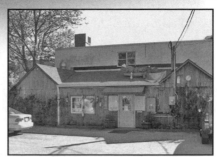

41 Oak Lane
Amagansett, NY 11930
631-000-0000
631-267-6700
fax 631-267-6709
stuartsseafood@optonline.net
stuartsseafood.com

Proprietors: Charlotte and Bruce Sasso

Directions: One block east of the Abraham's Path traffic light turn north. Located 1/2-block up on the left.

Season: Year-round.

Hours: 7 days a week, 9 A.M. to 6 P.M.; July and August 9 A.M. to 7 P.M.; January to March, closed Tue.

Products: Fresh local seafood, lobsters, soups, salads, clam pies. gourmet provisions, bread, desserts.

Special Events: Clambakes, barbecues, pig roasts, and other full-service catering.

About: One of the oldest fish markets on the East End. Local baymen deliver their catch daily.

Hampton Chutney

Amagansett Square, Montauk Highway
Amagansett, NY 11930
631-267-3131
hamptonchutney@verizon.net
hamptonchutney.com

Proprietors: Gary and Isabel MacGurn

Directions: East on Montauk Highway, Amagansett Square is located on the right after the Mobil station.

Season: Year-round.

Hours: Summer, 7 days a week, 10 A.M. to 7 P.M.; Fall and Spring, Wed. to Sun., 10 A.M. to 5 P.M.

Products: Fresh, natural cilantro, mango, peanut, curry, and tomato chutneys (and, in the fall and winter, pumpkin chutney).

About: Gary and Isabel MacGurn started making their fresh chutneys in 1995, selling them first to local Hamptons gourmet markets and then in New York City to Fairway, Zabars, Balducci's and others. In 1997, the couple opened their first dosa shop in Amagansett. The store is also a counter service restaurant with outside seating.

Gosman's Fish Market
West Lake Drive
Montauk, NY 11954
631-668-5645

Products: Local catches.

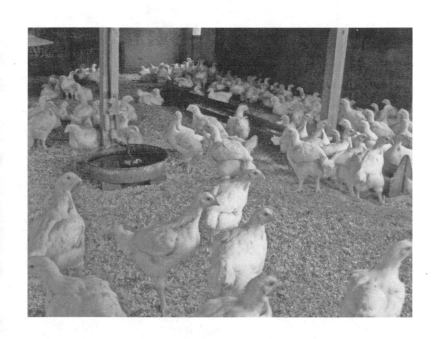

A Champion of Local, Regional Flavors

Bogo's Food Spa
27 Race Lane
East Hampton, NY

John Bogosian sells freshness. The speckled trout lettuce picked that morning, its oval leaves lightly splattered with maroon, a Jackson Pollack of greens, has it. In meats, he specializes in slow flavor, the kind that develops when an animal spends an extra nine to 12 months on the hoof grazing.

Knowledgeable customers who zero in on his tiny East Hampton shop at 27 Race Lane understand.

"They'll take all the freshest stuff. They go right by the organic lettuce from California, they'll go past everything else and they'll see only the lettuce that was harvested a few hours earlier down at the ECCO farm (East End Community Organic Farm). They just have radar for the local stuff. People know. The taste is there. The texture is there, and there's the look of it. People buy and eat food because it's beautiful." He thumbs the slim leaves of a tender Oak Leaf lettuce, its green fingers tinged with red, $1.99 a head.

Bogo's keeps slow-flavored, grass-fed, grass-finished, dry-aged beef from the New England Livestock Alliance (NELA) on hand frozen. It carries these in strip steaks, tenderloin, rib eye, hamburger meat and patties. There are also rich and meaty-flavored, low-fat bison burgers. Beef and bison patties average one-third pound and $2.25 each. New for the Fourth of July are kosher, natural beef hot dogs, $7.69 a pound.

It costs more, it takes longer to raise animals without antibiotics and growth hormones, and pesticides harbored in many animal feeds, particularly in chicken-feather meal or cottonseed feeds. Strip steaks run about $20 a pound. "About twice as much as you'd pay for regular steak," says Bogosian.

"The grass-finished meat is so lean, it's a completely different taste." It's created not only by slower growth, but by giving livestock elbow-room. Animals live outside excepting in severe weather. "People tell me that it tastes like meat used to taste," he says.

"It's very easy to overcook grass-finished steak," he warned the other day. "It doesn't have the fat. Cook it at a very high heat, rare on the inside." He was right. The first strip steak I tried overcooked in a flash, disappointing, dry. A second, cooked rare, had a level of flavor unknown in most meats today.

By ordering ahead customers can buy a wide range of fresh or frozen meats and fowl including Niman Ranch beef, pork and lamb, wild Alaskan salmon and halibut. Bogo's stocks the frozen fish, the wild salmon, $8.99 a pound. Orders for fresh and specialty items need to be placed by 5 p.m. Monday and Wednesday for next day delivery.

The seed for Bogo's might have been planted by his mother, an early feminist, who believed that a boy's place was in the kitchen. Bogosian began cooking family dinners at age seven. There were cans to open along with the day's bounty from clamming and fishing. "We were just beach rats in the summer," he smiled. But his palate was being shaped for fresh seafood. At one point he worked in a Rhode Island "weiner joint" which served some of country's best hot dogs. "They have a bite, you bite into them and they snap." Will Bogo's carry them? He shrugged, "They're probably not natural."

There was prep school, a stint as sous chef at Greenwich Village's Grove Street Cafe. Then he was sous chef at a little bistro near the French Mediterranean, an equidistant two-hour drive from the Spanish border and Marseille – a city with strong undercurrents of Moroccan flavors. He shopped for the bistro at local markets. Two-dozen oysters cost $3.00. "The local bounty was incredible. You had all the Pyrenees influences, the Basque region, the Spanish, the French, and it was all about fresh food, local herbs and spices."

Take a childhood of "austere" cooking, add to it an education in the fresh flavors of Southern Europe, work as an organic farmer and environmentalist, for business acumen toss in the creation of a successful internet-based software company, Runtime Technologies, with current clients like Chase Manhattan Bank and Compaq Computer, and you have the foundation for Bogo's Food Spa.

With the beginning of summer, the shop carries its own salads, guacamole, salsa, pesto, wraps and an organic line of hot soups.

And after Fourth of July hotdogs on Bogo's wheatfree, sprouted-grain buns, there's always the possibility of roasting a suckling pig.

—*Geraldine Pluenneke*

Cheese Alive with Flavor

Cavaniola's Cheese Shop
89 Division St.
Sag Harbor, NY

"When you get out to the East End, check out the new cheese shop in Sag Harbor," the manager of a top-rated New York metropolitan cheese shop urged an executive of chef Terrance Brennan's Artisanal Cheese Center. "A real city cheese shop way out there. And try one of their sandwiches," he continued.

"A cheese shop selling sandwiches?" His bemused listener's eyebrows and voice arched.

"Yes," the first sighed softly, "Cured sopressata sausage from Italy, marinated, roasted tomatoes and fontal cheese on a baguette."

Sandwiches elbowed in by accident. Cavaniola Gourmet Cheese Shop opened last season heading towards a summer peak of 160 cheeses, including 25 different blue cheeses, most artisanal products from small dairies, along with bottles of Verjus, comparable condiments and pastries. "Then one day I was making a sandwich for myself and someone wanted it, so I sold it to him. Someone else came in and wanted the same sandwich," says Michael Cavaniola. East End word-of-mouth spun sandwiches into bestsellers at $6.99 to $8.99.

Michael with his wife jumped careers as many have before them as a way to live full-time in Sag Harbor. For 15 years Michael worked as an architect, the last five designing interiors for offices of Bloomberg Ltd. around the world from France to Caracas. Working on the new 40,000 square foot Bloomberg headquarters in Manhattan, he met his future wife, Tracy, an interior designer who was selecting the carpet, fabric, and furniture.

But the architect's palate had been well-tutored in cheese from childhood. His parents owned the Cheese Shop of Ft. Lee, New Jersey for nineteen years. Michael and Tracy honeymooned tasting cheeses down Italy's Amalfi coast. On vacation the next year, they tasted their way down the California coast visiting dairies. When a "for rent" sign appeared one morning at 89 Division Street on Route 114, Tracy moved fast.

"Smelling and tasting is the best way to learn about cheese," says Michael. Everyone who enters the shop is offered tastes of whatever two or three cheeses sit on a cheese board on the counter. Most customers listening to the suggestions the Cavaniolas offer to those ahead of them in line – there is usually a line – ask for guidance. The confidence factor inspired by tasting the suggested cheeses often leads customers to buy far more cheese than they intended, and then they feel rather smug about it.

"With peaches?" asks Michael. He pulls out a luscious triple-creme Brillat-Savarin from Normandy. "Try this Roquefort from France. This particular dairy, Carles, is one of the best. It's a little expensive, $23.99 a pound. But it's almost like eating champagne." A respectable-sized chunk was $10.

There are the blues – from Spain and Italy, Stiltons from England, the multiple-award-winning "Roaring 40s" from Australia, top U.S. artisanal's blues: Bingham Hill from Colorado, Point Reyes Farm from California, Art Ludlow's Atlantic Mist from Bridgehampton.

For St. Patrick's Day the shop offered three Irish cheeses – a cheddar, a Cashel Blue from County Cork, and an herb-marinated goat cheese from Cavin. Plus the makings for Irish fondue – a recipe card and grated Irish cheese to combine with Guinness Stout from the beer store next door.

With the tastes, you hear something of the lore. One of Michael's favorites, Tarentise, an Alpine cheese, is made in Vermont in rare copper kettles. Another, a super-aged Gouda, is made by an 88-year-old dairyman west of San Diego. "We drizzle honey over this one. It's soooo good," Michael's face lights. The cheese shop's customer mix puts lie to the idea that good cheeses are an indulgence of the gourmet class. Eight and ten-year-olds, parents in tow, come in for their favorite caramel-toned goat cheese and Mecox Sunrise. Construction workers dash in for heady Irish cheddars and Stiltons. "If you're born out here you've developed a palate, clamming, fishing," reflects Michael.

Cavaniola cheese-keeping rules: Always serve at room temperature. Store cheeses at 45 to 50 degrees with high humidity; never enshrouded in plastic wrap. Instead, cover loosely with paper towel or aluminum foil. "For self-ripening cheese, only cover the edges of the cheese, never the bloomy white part," says Michael.

"The cheese is still alive," reminds Tracy.

"Is processed cheese alive?" a customer wonders.

"No," Michael shudders. "It's done for. It has no flavor. But it will last for years."

—Geraldine Pluenneke

The Mushroom Man

Open Minded Organics Mushrooms
Sag Harbor, NY

David Falkowski's interest in mushrooms all started with an auspicious encounter with the back-to-the-land bible known as The Humanure Handbook.

"Something turned on in my head," said Mr. Falkowski. "Something about the cycling of nutrients and elements on this planet."

Shortly after, Mr. Falkowski, a native of Bridgehampton, packed his bags for Olympia, Washington, to attend an immersion seminar with fungi guru Paul Stamets. He returned a certified "professional mushroom cultivator" with plans to launch the first commercial mushroom operation on the East End.

Things are moving fast. Both Mr. Falkowski and his fiancée Katherine Meyer left their previous jobs to work full time on the business. Several restaurants, including Robert's in Watermill, Bobby Van's in Bridgehampton, and Atlantica in Westhampton, are mixing the fungi in with their dishes. On a recent morning, when Mr. Falkowski delivered five pounds of Blue Oyster mushrooms to the Green Thumb Organic Market in Watermill, a woman claimed half the box before he had even set it on the counter.

"The product is beautiful," he said, inspecting a thick, shiny white Oyster mushroom. "You just don't see the same quality in the grocery store." (The mushrooms sell for $25 a pound at the Green Thumb, compared with $30 or more at most gourmet stores. "Ours are fresher and organic," said Mr. Falkowski, who often delivers the mushrooms within an hour of harvest.)

Everything begins on the microscopic level in the spawn laboratory that Mr. Falkowski built — a sterile, white-walled room about the size of a large closet where he stores and multiplies his mushroom spores. The room is equipped with a fan and filter that keeps out dust, insects, and airborne spores that might contaminate the seed stock. "This is the heart of it all," Mr. Falkowski said, who still feels like Dr. Who in his time-traveling vehicle Targus, when he slips on his sterile shoes, scrubs his hands with an isopropyl-alcohol solution, and shuts the door.

"This is our advantage over commercial mushroom operations in Pennsylvania and elsewhere," Mr. Falkowski explained. Growing premium mushrooms starts with high quality spores, which lose their vigor after a few generations. And they are expensive to buy. "The person who controls the spawn runs the company."

In a nutshell, Mr. Falkowski applies spores to a petri dish. Within a week, root-like mycelium have radiated outward and colonized the dish. Using an exacto knife, Mr. Falkowski transfers squares of the colonized medium into a glass jar of sterilized, organic rye grain — traces of fungicides can be lethal. The mycelia continue to grow and eventually make the glass jar look like it's stuffed with cotton balls.

At this point, the operation moves outside to a big boiling vat, where Mr. Falkowski sterilizes organically grown straw. Once the straw is cooled, in go the inoculated grains. Then, Mrs. Meyers unfurls a long plastic sac, holding the top open as Mr. Falkowski stuffs the straw in. "This is totally hands-on," he said. "No cheap labor. No machines."

The stuffed bags are tied at the top and hung from two-by-four rafters inside a climate-controlled greenhouse, where they resemble oversized sausages. Mr. Falkowski punctures the bags with a four-pronged arrowhead, creating spaces for the fruit — that is, mushrooms — to form. If the mix right, each sac should hold all the moisture and nourishment the mycelia need to take over the straw and yield several harvests or "flushes."

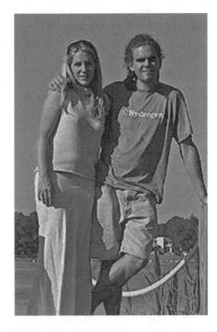

"Really all we're doing is helping nature along," said Mr. Falkowski. "Fungi are magicians of the soil." The first flush comes after about one month, followed by the next two ten days later. "It's only a month from attempt to result," he said. "That's better than the farmer who needs to wait the whole season."

The couple has run into a few problems, of course. They once had a catastrophe with gnats, which required them to sacrifice a large number of their growing columns, and hang yellow, sticky traps. "Mushroom growing is all about cleanliness," Mr. Falkowski said. "It's like farming in general. It's always going to be about something. This year is about the learning curve."

And they've progressed along the curve quickly. "Our yields from each sac have doubled since last month, and they're close to where we'd like them to be" a result of adding more inoculated grains to each sac and reducing the humidity in the greenhouse, Mr. Falkowski said. At 40 pounds a week, total supply still lags behind demand. "We need more sacs," Mrs. Meyer added. "Some chefs have been asking for 50 pounds a week."

In addition to Blue, White, and King Oyster mushrooms grown on straw columns, the couple is raising Shiitake, Chicken of the Woods, Hen of the Woods (also known as Maitake), and

Lion's Mane on logs. Eventually, Mr. Falkowski hopes to build a library of spores gathered from the many culinary mushrooms that grow wild on the East End.

Mr. Falkowski has cobbled together most of the mushroom-growing equipment himself, using salvaged wood and plastic, abandoned equipment, and frugal bidding on Ebay. Previously a landscaper, he uses the spent straw and wood chips from his mushroom growing as a nutrient rich compost on his collection of rare and exotic plants, including more than 30 types of edible berries. "One hand feed the other here," he said. "There's no such thing as waste." (Mr. Falkowski also sets up home mushroom beds for the gourmet gardener.)

As a wild and exotic food, mushrooms are enjoying a renaissance in culinary circles. Personally, Mr. Falkowski favors Shiitake — in omelettes, soups, salads, and stir-fries. And he raves about Mrs. Meyer's "barbecued oysters" recipe: Marinade Oyster mushrooms in olive oil, soy sauce, balsamic vinegar, and minced garlic, and grill. "It's the best finger-food you've ever had," Mr. Falkowski said.

Mrs. Meyer, who is training to be a natural foods chefs at the Natural Gourmet culinary school in New York, envisions an even broader gastronomic role. "In five years, we'd like to work with some of the wineries to arrange pairings," she said. "We can plan a new crop to be released with a wine. We'd like to be the one-stop shop for mushrooms on the East End."

But Mr. Falkowski thinks that most shoppers underestimate the health benefits of mushrooms. "They are not just a culinary treat," he said. "Think of them as a new generation of over-the-counter medicines."

Lion's Mane improves mental performance, he said. And Shiitakes strengthen our immune systems. A long list of antibiotics and antiviral medicines have been derived from fungi, and a recent study found that Oyster mushroom's help reduce bad cholesterol in the bloodstream.

Mr. Falkowski was recently checking the progress of an imminent crop, noting the tiny black-headed "pins" that will quickly expand into mature fruit. Adapting a common farm adage, he said: "I don't want to count my mushrooms before they pin."

—*Brian Halweil*

North Fork Farm Stands

Davis Peach Farm

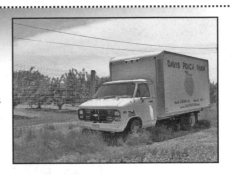

156 Hulse Landing Rd.
Wading River, NY 11792
631-929-1115
davispeachfarm.com

Directions: LIE exit 68 north to Rte. 25A. Take 25A east to Sound Avenue. Left on Sound Avenue to first light. Make left onto Hulse Landing Road.

Season: Early July to late October.

Hours: 7 days a week, 9 A.M. to 5 P.M.

Products: Over 100 varieties of u-pick peaches, plums, and nectarines; cider, pears, apples, apricots, over 50 varieties of plums. Also try plumcots, pruots, and apriums. A plumcot is a cross between a plum (50%) and an apricot (50%). A pluot is a cross between a plumcot and plum (75% plum/25% apricot). An aprium is 75% apricot and 25% plum!

Special Events: "Haunted hay rides" in October (call first).

About: Dave Davis, current owner of Davis Peach Farm, has farmed full time since 1950 on a farm originally owned by his father Archer. In 1992 "Pick Your Own Peaches" was established at the farm. In 2006, Dave planted 80 trees of "donut peaches," and today the farm features over 70 varieties of peaches.

John Condzella Farm

North Country Rd. (Route 25A)
Wading River, NY 11792
631-929-5058

Proprietor: John Condzella

Directions: Located one mile east of William Floyd Parkway on the north side.

Season: June to October.

Hours: 7 days a week, variable, usually 10 A.M. to 5 P.M., call in advance.

Products: Asparagus, strawberries, tomatoes, peppers, eggplant, broccoli, cauliflower cabbage, peas, beans. Pick your own.

May's Farm

Route 25A
Wading River, NY 11792
631-929-6654

Directions: LIE exit 68. Located one mile east of William Floyd Parkway on Rte. 25A.

Hours: 7 days a week, 9 A.M. to 6 P.M.

Products: Vegetables, flowers, plants, u-pick strawberries, peas.

Farmer Dan

3700 Middle Country
Road
Calverton, NY 11933
631-727-0149

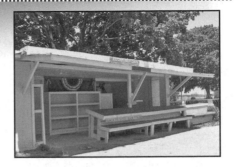

Proprietor: Dan Donahue Jr.

Directions: LIE Exit 71 North to Middle Country Rd. (Rte. 25). Make right. Farmstand is on left, next to Calverton Post Office.

Season: July to December.

Products: Potatoes, cauliflower, sprouts, cabbage, kale, collard greens, turnips, squash, pumpkins, gourds, carrots, beets, sweet corn, Indian corn, strawberry corn, string beans, tomatoes, peppers, eggplant, broccoli, apples, flowering kale, cucumbers, sweet potato.

Special Events: Dan wins about 25 vegetable awards at the Riverhead Country Fair each year and donates his potatoes for the Long Island Farm Bureau booth.

Lewin Farms

812 Sound Avenue
Calverton, NY 11933
631-929-4327
fax 631-929-6439
lewinfarms.com

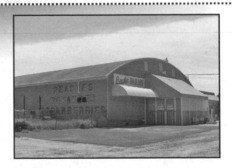

Proprietors: Dewey Lewin and sons

Directions: LIE exit 68 north (William Floyd Pkwy.) to very end, right on Rte. 25A, go to third traffic light, right on Sound Avenue. Farmstand is apx. 1/2 mile up the road on the right.

Season: Memorial Day weekend to first weekend after Thanksgiving, Christmas

Hours: 7 days a week, 9 A.M. to 5 P.M. For pick your own fields, call for availability.

Products: Full line of fresh fruits and vegetables. All fruits and vegetables grown on the farm are available as well as other produce locally grown. Pick your own: strawberries, peaches, tomatoes, peppers, eggplant, apples, pumpkins, and cut your own Christmas trees. Call first for availability and times.

About: Lewin Farms is a family owned and operated farm that has been on Long Island for three generations. It was the first pick your own farm on Long Island and continues this tradition.

Peconic River Herb Farm

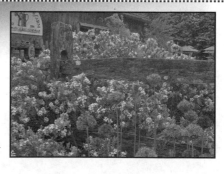

2749 River Road
Calverton, NY 11933
631-369-0058
fax 631-369-6179
prherbfarm@optonline.net
prherbfarm.com

Proprietor: Christina Spindler

Directions 1/4 mile north of LIE exit 71. Make left onto River Road and follow signs. Apx. 1/4 mile on left.

Season: April 1 to October 31.

Hours: April 1 to June 30, 9 A.M. to 5 P.M. daily; July 1 to October 31, 9 A.M. to 5 P.M. daily.

Products: Specialty retail plant nursery and scenic riverfront gardens. Spring: selection of herb, vegetable, and flower seedlings and their own honey. Summer/Fall: organic garlic, fresh and dried flower and herb bouquets. Available all season: their own line of certified organic dried herb and spice blends.

About: The plant selection at Peconic River Herb Farm has been continually upgraded over the past 20 years of growing both in their nursery and their extensive display gardens. Always featuring the latest cultivars as well as older "tried and true" selections that have proven to do well in the Long Island Zone 7 climate.

Rottkamp's Fox Hollow FarmStand

2287 Sound Ave.
Calverton, NY 11933
631-727-1786

Directions: LIE exit 71, north on Edwards Ave. to Sound Ave. (apx. 4 miles). Make right on Sound Ave. and travel 1/4 mile. Farmstand is located on the right side (south).

Season: June to October 31.

Hours: 9 A.M. to 5:30 P.M. everyday except Wed. and Sat. (9 A.M. to 4 P.M.).

Products: Their own sweet corn, lettuce, fruits, tomatoes, cakes, beans, summer and fall squash, yellow baby watermelons, pumpkins, corn stalks, corn maze U-pick pumpkins in October.

Windy Acre Farms

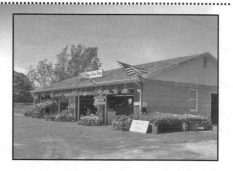

3810 Main Road
Calverton, NY 11933
631-727-4554

Directions: LIE exit 71. Make left at stop sign onto Edwards Ave. At light make left onto Route 25. Located 300 feet on right.

Season: May 1 to December 23.

Hours: 7 days a week, 9 A.M. to 6 P.M.

Products: Flowers, strawberries, corn, tomatoes, beans, peppers, pickles, eggplant, watermelons, jams, jellies, cauliflower, broccoli, pumpkins, squash.

Special Events: Roasted corn (July to October) on weekends only. Halloween pumpkin picking.

Andrews Family Farm and Greenhouses

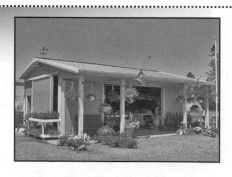

1038 Sound Ave.
Calverton, NY 11933
631-929-5963

Proprietor: Robert Andrews

Directions: LIE to exit 68; north to Route 25A east to Sound Ave. Located at corner of Sound Ave. and Hulse Landing Road.

Season: May to October 31. Also open in December with poinsettia, wreaths, and roping.

Hours: 7 days a week, 9 A.M. to 5:30 P.M.; in Dec., 9 A.M. to 4 P.M.

Products: Bedding plants, specialty annuals, hanging baskets and perennials (May and June). Fresh produce, roasted corn and cut flowers (July to October). U-pick pumpkins and field-grown mums (September and October). Poinsettias (December).

Special Events: Corn maze in October.

Fritz Lewin Farm

Corner of Sound Ave. and Edwards Ave.
Calverton, NY 11933
631-727-3346

Proprietor: Fred Lewin

Directions: LIE exit 71, left on Edwards Ave., go 4.5 miles. The field is located on the left-hand side.

Season: June to October.

Hours: 7 days a week, 9 A.M. to 5 P.M.

Products: Pick your own strawberries, tomatoes, peppers, eggplant, pumpkins, apples.

Will Miloski's Poultry Farm

4418 Route 25
Calverton, NY 11933
631-727-0239

Proprietor: Will Miloski

Directions: LIE Exit 71N to Route 25. Left on Route 25. Located two miles on right.

Season: February to December.

Hours: Wed. to Mon., 8:30 A.M. to 5:30 P.M. Closed Tuesdays.

Products: Locally grown turkeys; also other poultry and exotic game meats.

Anderson's Farmstand

Route 58
Riverhead, NY 11901
631-727-2559

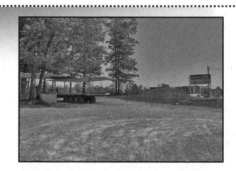

Proprietors: Richard and Faye Anderson

Directions: LIE exit 73 to Route 58 East, 2 miles on left side of Route 58.

Season: June 1 to October 30.

Hours: Weekdays, 9 A.M. to 6 P.M.; Sat. and Sun., 8 A.M. to 6 P.M.

Products: Strawberries, peas, corn, broccoli, cauliflower, onions, tomatoes, peaches, cucumbers, pickles, potatoes (red and white), peppers, cantaloupe, watermelon, beans, green & yellow squash, winter squash, pumpkins, gourds, cornstalks.

Special Events: U-pick strawberries in June.

Garden of Eve Organic Farm

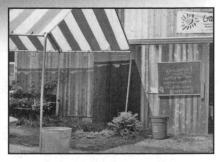

4558 Sound Avenue
Riverhead, NY 11901
631 722 8777
fax 631 727 6745
gardenofevefarm.com

Proprietors: Eve and Chris Kaplan-Walbrecht

Directions: Located on the north side of Sound Avenue at the intersection with Northville Turnpike.

Season: Memorial Day weekend to Thanksgiving.

Hours: 7 days a week, 10 A.M. to 6 P.M.

Products: Certified organic strawberries, pumpkins, heirloom tomatoes, sweet corn, lettuce, beets, carrots, many greens, herb plants, their own fresh-cut flowers, peppers, eggplant, garlic, and onions, and free-range eggs.

Special Events: Long Island Garlic Festival September 30 to October 1; U-pick pumpkins; see website for ongoing events.

About: Garden of Eve farm, founded in 2001, is dedicated to providing delicious organic vegetables, fruits and beautiful flowers and to "making changes in the world by living them." Garden of Eve's organic vegetables and flowers are available from farmstands in Riverhead, Long Island and in Brooklyn, and through Community Supported Agriculture shares.

Northville Farms

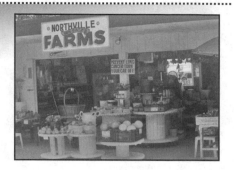

5333 Sound Avenue
Riverhead, NY 11901
631-722-3229
fax 631-722-4160

Proprietor: Gwen Gajeski

Directions: LIE exit 71. At stop sign, make left and go north 4 miles on Edwards Ave. Turn right onto Sound Ave., follow east to 1/2-mile past Church Lane. Farmstand is on south side (right).

Season: Memorial Day weekend to Thanksgiving.

Hours: 7 days a week, 9 A.M. to 6 P.M.

Products: Vegetables, fruits, flowers, baked goods. Yukon gold, russet, and green mountain potatoes, onions and shallots.

About: All season long, starting with the strawberries and ending with the pumpkins. Wheelchair accessible.

Ty Llwyd Farm

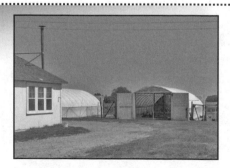

5793 Sound Avenue
Riverhead, NY 11901
631-722-4241
fax 631-722-4241
lizwines@hotmail.com

Proprietors: David and Liz Wines

Directions: Located just east of Manor Lane and west of Herrick's on Sound Ave.

Season: Year-round.

Hours: 7 days a week, 7 A.M. to 7 P.M.

Products: Free-range chickens, eggs, potatoes, vegetables and fruit in season. Occasionally, duck eggs are available.

About: This is a true family farm — husband, wife, and son — best known for their fresh brown eggs. All vegetables are grown on the farm with a minimum of sprays and pesticides. "Ty Llwyd" means "brown house" in Welsh. The farm has been in the family since 1870.

Briermere Farms

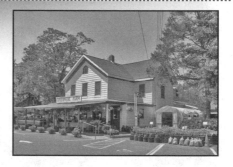

4414 Sound Avenue
Riverhead, NY 11901
631-727-2559
fax 631-722-8421
briermere@aol.com
briermere.com

Proprietor: Clark

Directions: LIE east to exit 73. Follow Rte. 58 east approximately 5 mi. Make left at traffic light onto Rte. 105 north to end (2 mi.). Make right onto Sound Ave. and quick left into driveway.

Hours: 7 days a week, 9 A.M. to 5 P.M.

Products: Apple butter, pure local honey, countless varieties of pies, jams, and jellies.

Reeve Farm

Sound Avenue
Riverhead, NY 11901
631-727-1095

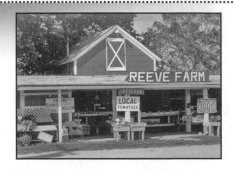

Proprietor: Richard L. Reeve

Directions: Located between Rte. 105 and Doctor's Path.

Season: May to November.

Hours: Thu. to Mon., 9 A.M. to 5 P.M. Closed Tue. and Wed.

Products: Vegetables, fruits, bedding plants, potted plants.

About: Debbie and Richard have run the farmstand for 35 years.

Mill Road Farms

Mill Road
Riverhead, NY 11901

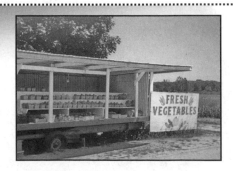

Products: Vegetables.

VerDerBer's Farmstand

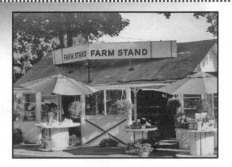

459 Main Road
Aquebogue, NY 11931
631-722-4388
fax 631-722-5422

Proprietor: Maria Verderber

Directions: Located 4/10 of a mile east of Rte. 105 on the Main Road in Aquebogue.

Season: October 1 to December 23.

Hours: Thu. to Sun., 9 A.M. to 6 P.M. (pumpkin picking on weekends through October).

Products: Vegetables, tomatoes, corn, cauliflower, broccoli, potatoes, squashes. Jarred jellies, dressings and more.

Special Events: Pumpkin picking, 10 acre corn maze, hayrides on weekends in October and Columbus Day.

Well's Homestead

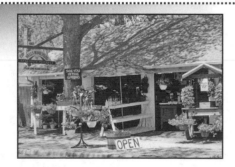

Rte. 25
Aquebogue NY, 11931
631-722-3796
fax 631-722-5422

Proprietor: Susan

Helen's Pumpkin Farm

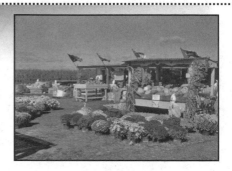

Union Avenue
Aquebogue, NY 11931

Bayview Farms and Market

891 Main Road
Aquebogue, NY 11931
631-722-3077
fax 631-722-7893

Proprietors: Brad and Lorraine Reeve and Sons

Season: April to November.

Hours: 7 days a week, 8 A.M. to 6 P.M.

Products: Asparagus, strawberries, sweet corn, spinach, tomatoes, broccoli cauliflower, brussels sprouts, roasted corn.

Special Events: U-pick strawberries in June.

Gabrielsen's Country Farm

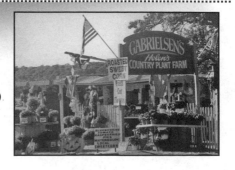

1299 Main Rd. (Rte. 25)
Jamesport, NY 11947
631-722-3259
fax 631-722-5922

Proprietor: George E. Gabrielsen

Directions: LIE last exit (exit 73). Continue east on Rte. 58. At traffic circle in Riverhead, stay on Rte. 58. Road changes to Rte. 25. Located about 4.5 miles from traffic circle on right-hand side.

Season: March 15 to December 24.

Hours: 7 days a week, 8 A.M. to 7 P.M.

Products: Flowering plants, hanging baskets, perennials, mums, sweet corn, strawberries, vegetables, pumpkins.

Special Events: Gabrielsen's Country Farm Fall Festival: September 11th to October 31 – corn maze, hay rides, pumpkins, restoration village.

Harbes Family Farm (Jamesport)

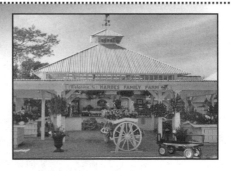

Main Rd. (Rte. 25)
Jamesport, NY 11947
631-722-2022
fax 631-298-1332
harbesfamilyfarm.com

Proprietors: Monica and Ed Harbes

Directions: From west: 495 east to last exit (Exit 73). East on Rte. 58. At the traffic circle in Riverhead, stay on Rte. 58. At Rte. 105, follow the "Farmstand Trail" sign east on Rte. 25, to our Jamesport location.

Season: July 1 to October 31.

Hours: 7 days a week, 9 A.M. to 6 P.M.

Products: Super-sweet corn, tomatoes, fruits and vegetables, roasted corn, baked pies, breads, jams, picnic area.

Special Events: Farm animals, school tours, Wild West maze (an 8-acre interactive maze September 4 to October 31, 9 A.M. to 5P.M. weekends), Fall Festival in Mattituck and Jamesport locations.

About: Harbes has expanded to two locations, and all eight of the Harbes children have taken an active part in farm operations, from plowing and harvesting the fields to running the farmstands.

Helen's Country Plant Farm

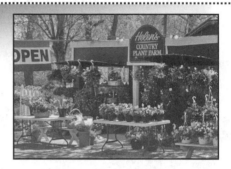

Main Rd. (Rte. 25)
Jamesport, NY 11947
631-722-5847
fax 631-722-5922

Bayview Market and Farms

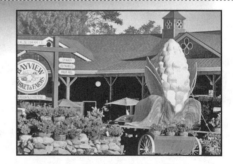

Main Rd. (Rte. 25)
Jamesport, NY 11947

Products: Vegetables.

Biophilia Organic Farm

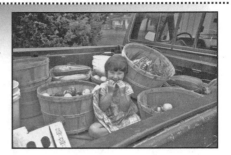

211 Manor Lane
Jamesport, NY 11947
631-722-2299

Proprietors: Phil and Mary Barbato

Directions: One-quarter mile north of Main Rd.

Season: April to December.

Products: Produce includes lettuce mix, tomatoes, potatoes, peppers (sweet and hot), beans, onions, garlic, squash, melons, kale, broccoli, sweet potatoes, eggplant, dill, basil, parsley, cilantro, oregano, sorrel, mint, flowers, and Christmas trees.

About: We are entering our seventh season farming organically on our 14-acre farm in Jamesport. Everything we grow is certified organic by NOFA-NY Certified Organic, LLC. We sell certified organic vegetable, herb, and flower plants in the spring. Our CSA members receive weekly shares of what we grow; our newsletter with farm news, recipes and ideas for the produce you receive; and special invitations for member-only events on our farm.

Golden Earthworm Organic Farm

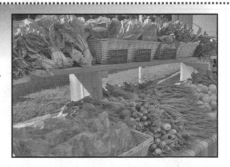

652 Peconic Bay Blvd.
Jamesport, NY 11947
631-722-23302
goldenearthworm.com

Proprietors: Matthew Kurek and James Russo

Directions: LIE exit 73; east on Rte. 58 through Riverhead; continue east into Jamesport; south on Washington Ave.; right at the first stop sign onto Peconic Bay Blvd. Located about a mile down the road on the right.

Season: May to November.

Hours: Fri. and Sat. 9 A.M. to 5 P.M.; Wed. 10 A.M. to 6 P.M.

Products: Over fifty different varieties of fruits and vegetables delivered to 17 CSA sites throughout Long Island and Queens, as well as local farmers' markets.

About: The Golden Earthworm Organic Farm CSA packs up a share of freshly harvested produce for every member and delivers it to a central pickup location once a week. The farm is nestled on 40 acres of pristine farmland protected by a land preservation program on the North Fork of Long Island, and was started in 1996 by Matthew Kurek, a chef turned farmer with a passion for growing top quality organic produce for the communities of Long Island.

Schmitt's Farm Country Fresh

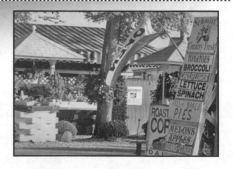

Main Rd. (Rte. 25)
Laurel, NY 11948
631-298-1991

Directions: LIE east to exit 73; Rte. 58 East through Riverhead; turns into Route 25; Approximately 5 miles east of Route 105.

Season: May 1 to October 31.

Hours: 7 days a week, 9 A.M. to 6 P.M.

Products: Fruits, flowers, vegetables, roasted corn, fruit pies.

Special Events: U-pick pumpkins and corn maze, September to October 7 days a week.

Harbes Family Farm (Mattituck)

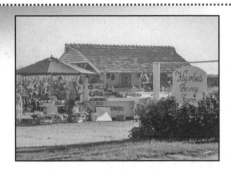

247 Sound Ave.
Mattituck, NY 11952
631-298-0800
fax 631-298-1332
harbesfamilyfarm.com

Proprietors: Monica and Ed Harbes

Directions: From west: 495 east to last exit (Exit 73). East on Rte. 58. At the traffic circle in Riverhead, stay on Rte. 58. Make a left onto Rte. 105, then a right onto Sound Ave. to visit our Mattituck location.

Season: May 1 to October 31.

Hours: 7 days a week, 9 A.M. to 6 P.M.

Products: Super-sweet corn, tomatoes, fruits and vegetables, roasted corn, baked pies, breads, jams, picnic area.

Special Events: Farm animals, school tours, Wild West maze (an 8-acre interactive maze September 4 to October 31, 9 A.M. to 5 P.M. weekends), Fall Festival in Mattituck and Jamesport locations.

About: Harbes has expanded to two locations, and all eight of the Harbes children have taken an active part in farm operations, from plowing and harvesting the fields to running the farmstands.

Hooterville Farms

Route 25
Mattituck, NY 11952

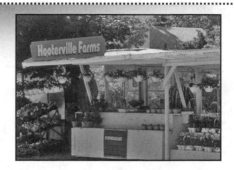

Wickham's Fruit Farm

28700 Main Road
Cutchogue, NY 11935
631-734-6441
fax 631-734-5454
wickhamsfruitfarm.com

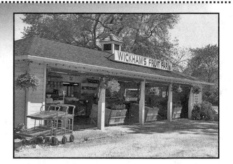

Proprietor: Prudence Heston

Directions: LIE to last exit (73). Take Rte. 58 east. Go straight for 15 miles. (Rte. 58 will become Rte. 25 along the way). Located on the right side of the road after first light in Cutchogue.

Season: May to December.

Hours: Mon. to Sat., 9 A.M. to 4 P.M. Closed Sundays.

Products: Rhubarb, asparagus, strawberries, plums, peaches, blackberries, field tomatoes, melons, corn, greens, apples, pears and pumpkins; baked goods, jams, pick-your-own cherries, raspberries, peaches and apples. The market offers homemade pies, donuts, jams, and other bakery items as well as apple cider in season.

Special Events: Tours and hayrides by appointment. Associated B&B.

About: Wickham's fresh produce is available both wholesale and retail through the roadside market in Cutchogue.

Satur Farms

3705 Alvah's Lane
Cutchogue, NY 11935
631-734-4219
info@saturfarms.com
saturfarms.com

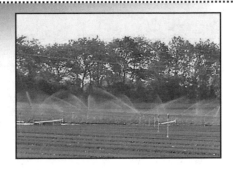

Proprietors: Paulette Satur and Eberhard Müller

Directions: From the west, get on Route 58/25 East. (Route 58 becomes Route 25 a few miles after you leave the LIE) As you approach Cutchogue, you'll pass Pellegrini then Gristina Vineyards. Take the first left after these wineries, which is Alvah's Lane. Satur Farms is located one mile ahead on the left.

Hours: No farmstand.

Products: Salad greens and specialty vegetables, sold only through Freshdirect.com and King Kullen stores on Long Island.

About: Satur Farms, owned by chef Eberhard Müller and his wife Paulette Satur, is dedicated to growing the finest vegetables and culinary ingredients, including specialty salads, leafy vegetables, heirloom tomatoes, root vegetables, and herbs. They are committed to farming according to organic standards, although not certified organic.

The Community Farm

5745 Alvah's Lane
Cutchogue, NY 11935

Proprietor: Denise Markut

Krupski's Pumpkin Farm

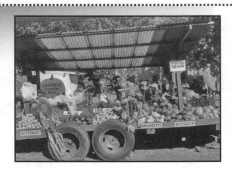

38030 Main Road
Peconic, NY 11958
631-734-6847

Proprietor: Al Krupski

Directions: LIE east to exit 73. Proceed 17 miles east on Route 25. Farm is located on south side of road.

Season: June 1 to December 1.

Hours: 7 days a week, 9 A.M. to 6 P.M.

Products: Sweet peas, sugar snap peas, organic lettuce, beets, Swiss chard, spinach, broccoli, cauliflower, Brussels sprouts, kale, cabbage, carrots, turnips, red, Yukon gold, and russet potatoes, white sweet corn, many tomato varieties, bell peppers, hot peppers, eggplant, cut flowers, sunflowers, hanging baskets, pumpkins, gourds, many winter squashes, corn stalks, broom corn, straw.

Special Events: Hayrides, haunted barn, haunted corn maze on weekends in the fall and for special events. Educational school tours in the fall.

About: Homegrown produce harvested daily.

Sang Lee Farms

25180 County Road 48
Peconic, NY 11958
631-734-7001
fax 631-734-7103
karen@sangleefarms.com
sangleefarms.com

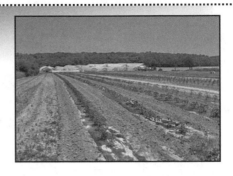

Proprietors: Fred and Karen Lee

Directions: LIE east to exit 73. Follow Route 58 to light at CR. 43 (Northville Tpke.). Turn left (north) onto Northville Tpke. and take to the end. Turn right onto Sound Ave. Located 14 miles down on the right.

Season: Year-round. Mail order available October 1 to May 1.

Hours: Summer: Mon. to Sat., 9 A.M. to 6 P.M.; Sun. 9 A.M. to 5 P.M. Winter: Thu. to Sat., 9 A.M. to 5 P.M., Sun. 11 A.M. to 5 P.M.

Products: Mesclun, baby spinach, baby arugula, other specialty baby greens, Asian vegetables, seasonal vegetables, 2 dozen varieties of heirloom tomatoes, cut/potted herbs, cut/potted flowers. Also, prepared dinner packs, veggie packs, specialty products including dressings, pestos, dips, cooking sauces, kimchees, salsas, pickled and preserved vegetables.

Special Events: CSA. Tours, tastings, cooking demonstrations, and classes. Call for a schedule.

About: Fred and his wife Karen operate the farm with their three children and staff growing more than 250 varieties of specialty vegetables.

Sep's Farm

7395 Route 25
East Marion, NY 11939
631-477-1583
fax 631-477-8305

Directions: From west: LIE Exit 73 to Route 25 East Marion. 1 mile east of Greenport on Route 25. From east: 5 miles west of Cross Sound Ferry on Route 25 between Orient and Greenport.

Season: May 1 to Thanksgiving.

Hours: 7 days a week, 8 A.M. to 5 P.M.

Products: Seasonally: asparagus, peas, rhubarb, strawberries, corn, tomatoes, lettuces, peppers, cucumbers, eggplant, string beans, flat beans, onions, cabbage, cauliflower, sprouts, broccoli, zucchini, beets, carrots, celery, winter squash, pumpkins, potatoes, cut flowers and more!

Latham Farms

Main Road
Orient, NY 11957
631-323-3701

Products: Vegetables.

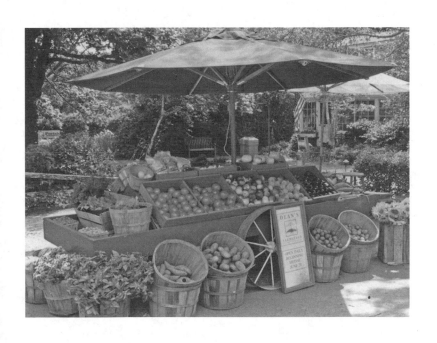

Garlic Jelly And
Easter Egg Chickens

Garden of Eve
4558 Sound Avenue
Riverhead, NY

Some who grow garlic say it absorbs the very character of the soil where it's planted, and eventually develops a unique flavor in the same way a great wine reflects its vineyard's specific swath of earth. Even before repeated plantings and the chemistry of terroir subtly influence its taste, newly-harvested varietal garlic is different than its bulk-grown brethren shipped cross-country. Peeled, its bulb is a pale cream, its flavor tangy.

On a recent Sunday, garlic and all manner of garlic products from North Fork producers could be tasted and bought at the Garden of Eve's first garlic festival. The organic farm in Riverhead offered "hard neck" German white garlics and more delicately-flavored "soft neck" Italian white, braids of the Italian garlic, and other garlics from Tom Stock's Sow-Love Reap-Joy Farm in Manorville. Catapano's Dairy Farm made a special herbed-garlic chevre for the occasion. Joan Bernstein sold a garlic jelly along with her other Paumanok Preserves. There were Sidor's North Fork potato chips, garlic breads from Baker's Bounty, Hans Lang's Chillin' and Grillin' marinades along with snacks of garlic-marinated chicken, garlic-cheddar sausage, and garlic curly fries. There was organic produce, such as heirloom tomatoes, cucumbers, squash, peppers, egg plants and flowers, grown by Eve Kaplan, the farm's Eve, and Chris Walbrecht, along with their garlic and eggs.

Since the days of Hippocrates in 460 BC, garlic has been revered for reputed therapeutic qualities. Today some research studies are suggesting it can kill bacteria, boost the immune system and even lower blood cholesterol. Kaplan says, "The better your soil, the better your garlic does," and conceivably its therapeutic potential. The acre of the farm where Kaplan and Walbrecht grew 1,000 pounds of *allium sativum* for the second year had been a hayfield untouched by herbicides or fertilizer in its prior life. "It had a lot of organic matter, a lot of worms." Organic farmers find worm holes thrilling. They are a tip-off to the richness of soil worms help create. "The soil is especially important because its nutrients are going directly into that garlic root, a tuber. It's the way the plant stores up nutrients for the next year," says Kaplan.

Until the mid-seventies virtually all widely distributed garlic – first introduced as a crop in the United State in the early 1900s – was a "soft neck" variety commercially produced in Gilroy, California. It's the garlic you usually find in supermarkets, though worldwide there are 600 different sub-varieties of garlic.

Then Alice Waters held her first garlic dinner at Chez Panisse in Berkeley, and though no one in the restaurant can remember exactly when, word spread of the extraordinary flavors Waters conjured up that night with garlic. Garlic growers from Texas to upstate New York have told me that reports of the menu enticed them to jump careers. "That dinner was the first American garlic festival," one said.

Today there are close to 100 garlic festivals in the US, some drawing attendees from across the country, others like Garden of Eve's introducing local products to the local area. Thousands of impassioned growers of varitial garlic with opinions as strong as raw garlic breath debate what soils to use to coax richer and deeper garlic taste out of the ancient bulbs. But one thing they uniformly praise – worm holes.

This was the first year Kaplan and Walbrecht, who farm a total of 15 acres, operated a highway stand at Garden of Eve in Riverhead, selling produce and plants. For three years they had sold their organic produce at farmers' markets in Tribeca, Greenpoint in Brooklyn, Port Washington, and the Thursday Riverhead market.

The festival also included a "petting zoo" in which children could pet chickens and ducks. "You'd be surprised how many kids have never touched a chicken or a duck," said Kaplan.

"Have you ever petted a chicken?" a visitor asked suspiciously with memories of the farm's flock of 250 chickens and several dozen ducks scuttling hastily free from her shadow.

"Yeah, of course, all the time. They're very tame," Eve replied blandly. "They're frightened at first. But there will be an adult to help," she added.

In an unusual twist, parents may have heard their children begging them to buy a half-dozen fresh organic eggs for $2. Almost half the laying chickens are Araucana, "called the Easter Egg chicken," explained Kaplan, who adds their eggs are lower in cholesterol than normal chickens. The Araucanas are also more creative. The same hen may lay a pink-tinted egg one day, a blue the next, and on another a green. I guess to these birds, every day is Easter!

—*Geraldine Pluenneke*

Sang Lee Farms

Sang Lee Farms
25180 County Road 48
Peconic, NY

"If there's anything I've learned it's change or die," said Fred Lee. He has grown wheat for making bread. (Good crop, but no market.) He's planted a grove of Asian pears. (Worked, but the harvest largely went to family and friends.) "If I haven't changed or re-evaluated something, I'm standing still."

But step into the shop at Sang Lee Farms in Peconic on the North Fork, and you will see the results of lots of experiments that did work. In fact, you might think you have entered a time warp, fast-forwarding to summer. The shelves are teaming with color, filled with items that most other Long Island farms won't harvest until July or August.

Baskets overflow with leeks, radishes, carrots, beets, onions, scallions, potatoes, garlic, and tomatoes (cherries and Beefsteak), as well as more predictable choices like spinach, mesclun, and asparagus. There's a cooler filled with a dizzying assortment of bagged Asian greens: Stir-fry combo pack, Baby Bok Choy mix, Pea Shoots, Shanghai Choy, Nyu Choy Sum, Guy Lon, Mizuna, and Tatsoi.

"Right now, we're ahead, but not for long," Mr. Lee said, who is soft-spoken with perfect diction. (During the day, he will variously speak English, Spanish, or Cantonese.) He sports a "Sang Lee Farms" cap and a neat, salt-and-pepper mustache.

Customers stream in and out of the shop, buying potted flowers for their garden or greens and stir-fry sauce (also made on the farm) for dinner. But, while the Lee family has been farming here for over sixty years, this bustling operation is relatively new. "It's been an evolution," Mr. Lee said.

In the 1970s, when Mr. Lee took over the family farm that his father and uncle began in the 1940s, it grew roughly a dozen Asian vegetables like Chinese cabbage, bok choy, and Napa cabbage to supply Chinatowns from New York to Toronto. It was a reliable niche market. But that didn't last.

"As soon as the supply came on from other regions or off-shore, our prices began to fall," Mr. Lee recalled. The family was cultivating 550 acres in Long Island and Florida, ramping up the volume as the profits fell. "We asked 'What else can we grow'," said Mr. Lee.

Some neighbors and drive-by shoppers began asking if they could buy some of the greens that were being shipped to restaurants and supermarkets in brightly colored "Fresh-Lee-Cut" boxes. Karen, Fred's wife, set up a self-serve stand shaded by an umbrella on the roadside. The stand sold out almost hourly. "When the weather got cold, we had to move it into a corner of the garage where farm works used to eat their lunch," said Carol Betterman, a friend and neighbor who started working at the farm around this time.

Today, this white-washed farmstand on County Road 48, open 7-days-a-week all year, has two cash registers and accounts for some 70 percent of Sang Lee's sales. The family has sold the Florida acreage and scaled down to the 23-acre family farm in Peconic and 40-acres it leases nearby. The farm raises over 250 different varieties of vegetables, herbs and flowers, including 35 varieties of tomatoes. "The mesclun mix alone contains more species than we used to raise," Mr. Lee said.

The adjustment was good for business, but it hasn't always been smooth. "Before I would put in 10 acres plantings at a pop. Now, I'm lucky if I plant one-tenth of an acre," Mr. Lee said. He zips around the farm on a battery powered golf cart, part of a fleet of four that he uses to move seedlings or harvested crops. "We're not harvesting tractor-trailer loads any

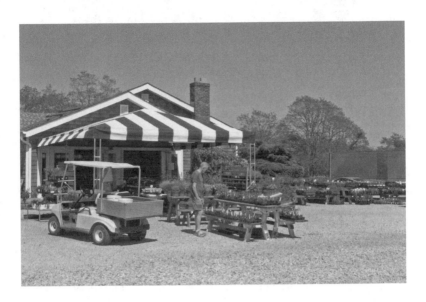

more, and we don't have to worry about oil changes and air filter servicing."

The family farm also includes "36,000 square feet under poly," as Mr. Lee describes his greenhouses, which have become a central facet of the operation. The three large greenhouses are heated, and during the last few hard winters, the fuel bills in January and February made Lee question the operation. "I literally set the thermostat at 32 degrees to keep the greens from freezing," Mr. Lee said

But, by March, Sang Lee has a crop roughly sixty days ahead of anyone else. "It allows me to get a jump on the season," Mr. Lee said, weeding in one of his greenhouses surrounded by trellised tomato, French radishes, and seemingly endless rows of tiny lettuce leaves in a rainbow of green and red. Getting customers early might mean keeping them through the entire year.

A final stage in the farm's evolution is a commercial kitchen connected to the farmstand, where Mrs. Lee and Mrs. Betterman turn surplus produce into dressings (ginger scallion, Asian vinaigrette, toasted sesame, and citrus), pestos (cilantro, basil, arugula, and spinach), and dips (herb garlic and ginger scallion). "Actually, Fred's step-father was doing a stir-fry demo with our greens and everyone started asking what he put in," said Mrs. Betterman.

In the jargon of agricultural officials, Sang Lee farm is a model of "value-added agriculture." By turning a $2 bunch of basil into a $6 jar of pesto, the farm is "holding onto more of the food dollar."

For Mr. Lee, it's just common sense. Being able to respond to feedback from customers is "my only advantage over distant shippers in California, Mexico or offshore," Mr. Lee said. Every year, Mr. Lee introduces several new varieties of flowers or veggies, whether its yellow carrots or Mexican sunflowers, to "keep the product mix changing," he said. "Come this fall, we'll sit down and we'll ask how we can improve on even those things that worked well."

The farm recently started selling kimchi, and will soon roll out a carrot soup. "That's them guys," Mr. Lee said in a feigned farmer's drawl, referring to several women in the kitchen. One of them shouted back, "But you grow it!"

—*Brian Halweil*

Saying Cheese

Catapano Dairy Farm
33705 North Road
Peconic, NY

Words that leap to mind while tasting Michael and Karen Catapano's goats milk yogurt have nothing to do with health. Decadent is more like it. "Outrageous, dense," pronounced an East Hampton retailer after tasting a lone spoonful. The Catapano's fetas and chevres are serious cheeses, bespeaking pleasure, forget well-being. A new aged brie-style blue cheese has unexpected fullness. It is rich with a dense aftertaste.

For cheese-maker Michael Catapano, an M.D., impressions of indulgence count.

"To me it's a taste treat, not something I eat as a medicine," he says. His wife Karen, a former nurse, contradicts, "I see the other side of it." She numbers some of the health benefits of goats' milk products that seem to benefit the lactose intolerant, and people with skin and digestive problems. "Overall, it's a more nutritious product than cows' milk because its fat globules are very tiny. It's very high in protein, like human milk, high in essential amino acids, and has a higher evolved form of carotene, a precursor of Vitamin A."

The Catapanos, on their thriving dairy farm on Sound Avenue in Mattituck, are part of a new breed of farmers, often highly-educated in other fields and drawn to the land after successful first careers. Karen, a nurse with a masters degree in gerontology, ran a cardiac rehabilitation center at Southampton Hospital for eight years before creating a $2-million department, The Center for Community Health and Wellness. In 1995, Michael's career in emergency medicine brought him to the emergency department at Southampton Hospital and into Karen's orbit. He now works four ten-hour days with the Walk-in-Medical Center in Wainscott, makes cheese for another three ten-hour days, and somehow has found time to write a murder mystery.

Karen grew up surrounded by animals in Oyster Bay, on Nassau County's North Shore. By the time Michael met her she was and still is breeding Ragdoll and Siberian cats and cocker spaniels. Michael, whose grandfather raised goats in Italy before he farmed in Brooklyn, spent his first five years on a produce farm.

"I remember hauling crates of cauliflower up on the truck," he says.

His family now runs Catapano Farms, a Southold nursery. In 2003, the couple learned the Mattituck dairy was for sale.

"We decided to buy the farm, change our life and live here," said Karen.

But first they tested out their affinity for goats with a two-week immersion on a 30-goat dairy farm. There they absorbed every detail of goat care and cheesemaking, just like goats' milk absorbs every flavor in a goat's diet. This kind of precision and thoroughness appears to run through everything they do.

Today they have 30 "milkers" of their own, eight babies, and a pending application as an organic producer. Initially, they failed to anticipate the staggering expense of producing cheeses with the level of flavor they wanted. After a $200,000 startup investment, they spent half again as much on the unexpected. Everything was expensive.

"Something like a little ladle is," Karen's voice rising in surprise, "$500! Stainless steel, no welding."

The Catapanos found "milkers" to fulfill their flavor profile and have replaced all but three of their original goats. Many are registered show goats, costing $500 each. Their cheeses are made by blending milk from a breed with high fat content, from another with extra sweet milk, from two with prolific volume.

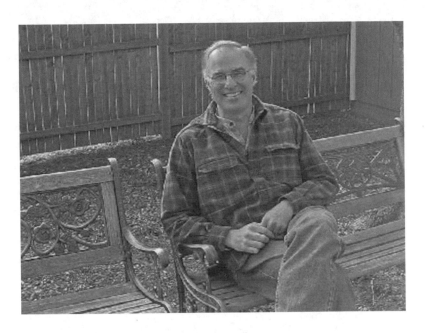

The farm's fetas and chevres are available in top East End markets. You can sample them at The Cheese Shop in Southampton and Mattituck, The Green Thumb in Water Mill, Round Swamp Market in East Hampton, Cavaniola in Sag Harbor, at Sang Lee's in Peconic, at Manhattan's Union Square greenmarket, and at some vineyards.

But to taste sinful yogurts, you have to visit their North Fork shop at 3985 Sound Ave. in Mattituck. There you'll find fetas, plain chevres, herb-rolled chevres, cheddar-style and air-dried basket cheeses, and whole milk ricotta. There is goats' milk fudge, goats' milk butter and a goat cheese cookbook. Children can feed the baby kids in their pen right by the shop.

There are also full-fat goats' milk soaps with surprisingly soft-silky suds, so perhaps there is something to the legend that its liposomes help seal moisture in the skin.

You can buy a picnic to go for a visit to a local vineyard for $20 for two. It includes plates, cups, utensils, napkins, crackers, fudge and any two cheeses. And the future? Says Karen, "Maybe Michael will make more yogurt so we can sell it other places." Despite his full schedule, with Michael's track record, it seems likely he'll achieve this goal.

—*Geraldine Pluenneke*

North Fork Purveyors

Crescent Duck Farm

Edgar Ave.
Aquebogue, NY 11931
631-722-8000
fax 631-722-5324

Proprietor: Douglas Corwin

Directions: Call ahead. Also sell at Bayview and Wells Farmstands.

Season: Year-round.

Hours: Mon. to Fri., 9 A.M. to 5 P.M.

Products: Ducks.

About: Founded in 1908 by Doug Corwin's great-grandfather, Crescent Duck Farm is mainly a wholesale operation but you can buy direct from them. Please call ahead.

Braun Seafood Co.

Main Road
Cutchogue, NY 11935
631-734-7770

Hours: Sun. to Thu., 9 A.M. to 6 P.M.; Fri. to Sat. 9 A.M. to 8 P.M.

Products: Local catches.

Southold Fish Market

Main Road
Southold, NY 11971
631-765-3200

Products: Local catches.

Alice's Fish Market

Monsell Place
Greenport, NY 11944
631-477-8475

Products: Local catches.

Catapano Dairy Farm

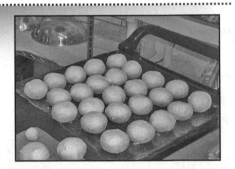

33705 North Road
Peconic, NY 11958
631-765-8042
catapanodairy@aol.com
catapanodairyfarm.com

Proprietors: Karen and Michael Catapano

Season: April 15 to November 1.

Hours: 7 days a week, 9 A.M. to 5 P.M.

Products: Fresh goat cheese and yogurt. Pure, 100% goat milk skin-care products.

Special Events: Tour groups welcome, by appointment.

About: Received the first place award for their chevre cheese from The American Cheese Society in 2005. (The American Cheese Society considered one of the world's most influential and prestigious competitions in recognizing the art of artisanal and specialty cheesemaking.)

North Fork Chips

2010 Oregon Road
Mattituck, NY 11952
631-298-8631
northforkchips.com

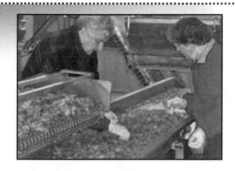

Proprietor: Martin Sidor

Products: North Fork Chips has been growing potatoes on their family farm in Mattituck for three generations. They kettle-cook their potatoes to make super-crispy chips with a hearty potato flavor.

Up-Island FarmStands

Youngs Farm: The Annex

Hegeman's Lane
Old Brookville, NY 11545
516-626-3955
fax 516-626-3805.

Proprietors: Jo-Hana and Paula

Directions: First right north of the intersection of 25A and route 107. Take Hegeman's Lane 1/2 mile on left.

Season: February 7 to December 23.

Hours: Tue. to Sat., 10 A.M. to 5 P.M.; Sun., 11 A.M. to 4 P.M.

Products: Locally grown products or grown on our farm: corn, tomatoes, squash, peaches, strawberries, raspberries, beans, peppers, homemade pies, breads, soups, jams, chicken pot pie, country gift shop.

About: One of the last remaining farms in Nassau.

Mediavilla Orchards

1527 East Jericho Turnpike
Huntington, NY 11743
631-423-4794

Proprietor: Mary Pombo

Directions: Located 1/4 mile east of Deer Park Avenue.

Season: August 15 to Thanksgiving.

Hours: Tue. to Sun., 9:30 A.M. to 5 P.M.

Products: Apples, peaches, plums, pears, cider, jams, jellies, grapes, chestnuts.

Sophia Garden

555 Albany Ave.
Amityville, NY 11701
631-842-6000 ext. 307
sophiagarden@aol.com
members.aol.com/sophiagardens

Proprietors: Sisters of St. Dominic

Directions: No farmstand.

Season: May to November.

Products: The garden has 110 member families and grows a wide variety on less than two acres. They are in their tenth year. Next year they will add an additional acre.

Special Events: CSA. Concerts and lectures.

Richters Orchard

Pulaski Road
Northport, NY 11768
631-261-1980

Proprietors: Louis and Andrew Amsler

Directions: Located on the north side of Pulaski Road, 1.3 miles west of Sunken Meadow Parkway.

Season: August to May.

Hours: 7 days a week, 9 A.M. to 5:30 P.M.

Products: Apples, peaches, cider mill, pumpkins.

Johnson's Farm

123 Cedar Road
East Northport, NY 11731
631-266-1822
hojofarms@aol.com

Directions: Jericho Tpke. (Rte. 25) to Larkfield Road; north 1 mile to Cedar Road. Located 1/4 mile east on Cedar Road.

Season: April 15 to October 1.

Hours: 7 days a week, 9 A.M. to 6 P.M.

Products: Fruits, vegetables, plants, bedding plants, flowers, hanging baskets.

Brightwaters Farms and Nursery

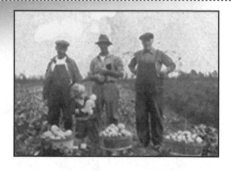

1624 Manatuck Blvd.
Bay Shore, NY 11706
631-665-5411
fax 631-665-0223
brightwatersfarms.com

Directions: LIE exit 53 south, follow pumpkin signs or Southern State Parkway to exit 42 south, follow pumpkin signs.

Season: September 24 to October 30.

Hours: 7 days a week, 10 A.M. to 5 P.M.

Products: Pumpkins, sweet corn, squash, cucumbers, tomatoes, gourds, honey, cider, apples, fresh baked goods.

Special Events: Every weekend: a banjo country band, roasted corn, snack patch, u-pick pumpkins, fall festival, pony rides, farmers playland, hayrides.

About: Brightwaters Farm has been in existence since the late 1600s. The land was purchased from the King of England by the Phelps family, the farms' original founders.

Borella's Farmstand

485 Edgewood Avenue at 25A
St. James, NY 11780

Directions: LIE exit 56 north approximately 5 miles (Route 111 North) to Route 25A east; Left onto Edgewood Ave. Located 1/2 mile on right side.

Season: Easter to Thanksgiving.

Hours: 7 days a week, 9 A.M. to 6 P.M.

Products: Flowering annuals and perennials, roses, shrubs, herbs, vegetable plants, hanging baskets, specialty planters, cut flowers, fresh fruits and vegetables in season, autumn decorations, mums, flowering cabbage and kale, u-pick pumpkins, cornstalks, apples, cider, freshly baked pies, jams, candied apples, Spring 2005 newly planted vineyard.

BB GG Farm and Nursery

625 North Country Road
St. James, NY 11780
631-862-9182
fax 631-862-9075

Proprietor: William Borella

Season: Easter to Christmas.

Hours: 7 days a week, 8 A.M. to 6 P.M.

Products: Nursery plants, annuals, perennials, fruits, vegetables, mulch, compost.

Special Events: Hay rides, corn maze.

Deer Run Farms

282 South Country Rd.
Brookhaven, NY 11719
631-286-7299
deerrun7@optonline.net

Proprietors: Robert and Janet Nolan

Directions: Sunrise Hwy. to Station Road (exit 56). South on Station Road approximately 2 miles to South Country Road. Left at the light and proceed East on South Country Road for apx. 1 mile. Farmstand is located on the right.

Season: Early June to Thanksgiving.

Hours: Thu. to Sun., 10 A.M. to 6 P.M., Weekends only after Labor Day.

Products: A wide selection of farm fresh fruits and vegetables, many varieties of home grown lettuce, cabbage, spinach, sweet corn, tomatoes, local berries, local honey, jams, and preserves, local goat cheese from Catapano Dairy and Holey Moses Gourmet Fruit Pies.

Special Events: Wholesale many varieties of lettuce, spinach, cabbage, escarole and chicory.

Hamlet Organic Farm (HOG)

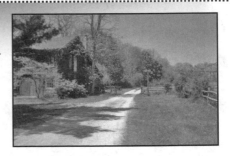

Brookhaven, NY 11719
631-286-7068
*mail@
hamletorganicgarden.org*

Proprietors: Jill Garrick and Sean Pilger, managers

Season: May 15 to October 31.

Products: Over 350 varieties of vegetables, herbs, fruits and flowers, including lettuce, broccoli, tomatoes, carrots, as well as specialty greens, heirloom melons and tomatoes, and fresh culinary herbs.

About: Hamlet Organic Garden is a community farm located in Brookhaven hamlet. Since 1996, they have grown certified organic vegetables, herbs, and cut flowers on a 5 acre farm field. Most of the farm production is sold as shares in a community supported agriculture (CSA) project. A share provides between 5 and 18 pounds of produce and a bouquet of flowers each week from mid-May until the end of October. Certified organic by NOFA-NY.

Little Red FarmStand

210 Yaphank–Middle Island Road
Yaphank, NY 11980
631-205-9579

Proprietor: Bob Borella

Directions: LIE exit 66 (Sills Road) to Middle Island–Yaphank Road. Located next to Middle Island Golf Course.

Season: July 1 to October 31.

Hours: 7 days a week, 9 A.M. to 6 P.M.

Products: Sweet corn, lettuces, tomatoes, peppers, squashes, cabbage, string beans, cauliflower, local fruits in season.

Special Events: U-pick pumpkins, corn maze, hay rides, roasted corn, candied apples, fall products, all Halloween needs. Buses welcome (call for appointment).

Pumpkin Patch Farm Stand

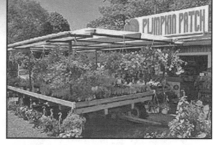

142 Long Island Ave.
Yaphank, NY 11980
631-924-7444
fax 631-924-5178
pumpkinpatchfarmstand@juno.com
pumpkinpatchfarmstand.com

Proprietors: Don and Pat Allen

Directions: LIE exit 66 north. Located 500 feet on corner.

Season: May 1 to Thanksgiving.

Hours: 7 days a week, 9 A.M. to 6 P.M.

Products: Roasted peppers, corn, lettuce, fruit, tomatoes, flowers, perennials, annuals, cheesecake, pies, honey, bread.

About: A farmstand run by a third generation, native Long Island farm family. The business started more than twenty-five years ago on forty dollars worth of Mother's Day flowers and an old wire reel not far from their present location. Today they have a small open-air farmstand and greenhouses for the hanging baskets, bedding plants and perennials that are sold all season long.

Lenny Bruno Farmstand

Wading River Road
Manorville, NY 11949
631-549-2029

Proprietor: Lenny Bruno

Directions: LIE Exit 69 South. The stand is right there.

Season: June to November.

Hours: 7 days a week, 9 A.M. to 6 P.M.

Products: Strawberries, sweet corn, eggplant, tomatoes, peppers. Just about everything except lettuce.

Special Events: Pick your own tomatoes, eggplants, peppers, beans starting in August.

About: Brunos have been farming in the area for more than sixty years, over three generations.

Unusual Spuds

Marilee Foster
Tiger Spud Potato Chips
Sagaponack, NY

Armed with a spading fork, Marilee Foster dug some potatoes that are unlike any other the family raises in Sagaponack.

She leaned into the trough between potato rows, loosening the soil below. She bent down to unearth a cluster of dark green stalks, a dozen or so red-skinned spuds dangling below. She dusted one off, and, holding a nearby shovel with the handle in the ground, severed the potato on the shovel blade. She inspected the pinkish core and seemed satisfied.

"It's definitely a trial run," Ms. Foster said, as she looked over this lush field on the east side of Sagg Main Street. "They have all done pretty well. It's not a bad crop."

Not bad, considering that the field sustained an infestation of potato beetles, pervasive rumors of potato blight, and an unusually dry spring.

And, not to mention that Ms. Foster raised the crop in compliance with federal organic standards. No chemical fertilizer touched the soil. No synthetic pesticides dusted the plants.

"Twenty years ago, farmers would have laughed at us," Ms. Foster said. "Plenty of people laugh at us today."

Federal standards released in 2002 encouraged more farmers and shoppers to consider organic foods. Organic crops generally fetch a higher price for the farmer, who can also reduce costs — and health care worries — by avoiding expensive pesticides. In the case of Long Island potato growing, a historic decline in potato beetle pressures — partly because so many potato farms have gone out of business — also helped.

As elsewhere, many East End farmers remain skeptical. Some might even consider organic farming a liability. "They are growing right next to the fields that feed our farm," Ms. Foster said. "It could be a little festering disease hole."

For the last two decades, this one-acre "pilot" plot served as a horse pasture. That means no chemical residues, which can prolong the organic certification process.

But twenty years of pounding horse hooves also packed the top layer, requiring Ms. Foster's brother Dean to "break it open" by dragging a plow and disker across the field several times, before shaping airy mounds for the spuds.

Underneath, the Bridgehampton Loam — so revered that it occupies the top position in the United States Department of Agriculture's list of soils — was still intact. "What's better for growing something organically than the most fertile land you've got?," Ms. Foster asked.

The field holds six varieties of potatoes, with names like Caribé, Island Sunshine, and All-Blue. All are more colorful, and less uniform, than the "big, old white potatoes" that make up most of the Foster fields. A variety called, Prince Hairy, lines the perimeter.

"It's supposed to be naturally potato beetle resistant," she added. "It's not."

At times, the venture has also inspired some difficult intro-spection. "We know that all the potatoes we grow are wholesome and safe," Ms. Foster said. "So what does it mean that we can't spray certain things on this plot?"

And using organically approved compounds doesn't come without worry. At least one fungicide approved for use on organic potato farms contains the same active ingredient, albeit in smaller doses and with fewer additives, as a fungicide the Fosters use elsewhere on the farm. "The pollution from cars driving by is probably worse that what we spray," she said.

The day she was spraying an approved product called Entrust, derived from a soil dwelling bacterium that is toxic to certain leaf beetles, thousands of dragonflies were hatching in the one-acre potato patch. "I said, please don't let this kill them," Ms. Foster remembers. It didn't.

The handful of other organic farmers on the East End have been generous with advice. Steve Storch of Natural Science Organics in Watermill sprayed the field with compost tea — a microbe-rich stew of manure and decomposing plants — followed by a plant-fortifying concoction made from nettles, equisetum and silica. And Mr. Foster injected additional compost tea into the soil when he cultivated the field for weeds.

Outside of the field, Ms. Foster has learned a bit about the economics of organic farming. "The seed is ten times as expensive," she said. "And everything else is about that much more."

Organic certification also requires piles of paperwork. The Fosters must steam-clean all of their plows, harvesters, and sprayers, before taking them onto the organic acre.

After a marathon session of pencil pushing, Ms. Foster sent her forms to the Northeast Organic Farming Association, the certifier for New York's organic farms. Several weeks later, she was startled to receive a request for additional information. "I can't even account for the amount of time I've spent record keeping," she added.

Still, the Fosters are considering certifying several adjacent acres of land as organic, and using them as a sort of "organic" arm of their operation.

"It's plain old diversification," she said. "I don't see it as organic versus conventional. It's almost like a whole other vegetable. I do find it sort of exciting, because for sometime I've felt the revolution is here, and we're not going to make do selling potatoes at $5 a hundredweight. We want a niche product that we don't have to deal with tons of."

Even at $4 a pound, the potatoes, the only "organic" item for sale on the Sagg Main farmstand strip, have been flying off the shelf. (Ms. Foster, who recently set-up a micro-chippery on the farm, hasn't yet turned any of the organic spuds into chips, although an organic inspector recently certified the facility.)

If she can't sell the whole crop through the farmstand or to restaurants and groceries, she's considering a few weeks of dig-your-own potatoes in the fall. "People dig them from us all the time," she said.

Maybe this time they'll pay.

—Brian Halweil

The Funky Chickens of Amagansett

Quail Hill Community Farm
Side Hill Lane and Deep Lane
Amagansett, NY

It's 8 AM and the chicken coop at Quail Hill Farm in Amagansett is restless.

Josh May, a farm apprentice, opens the gate and a few stir crazy birds leave to start their day. Josh claims the chickens like his voice. "But I talk to anything so I'm probably not the best person to ask," he confesses. Josh collects the eggs laid the night before, replenishes the feeder, and lays new sawdust into the wood cubbies where the hens nest.

As the birds come out of the dappled and dusty coop and into the cool sunlight, the full dimensions of this motley crew become clear.

Among 45 hens (and one fortunate rooster) there are fifteen distinct breeds. Together they look like extras from the Muppet Show with floppy appendages and jarring colors.

The cast includes Golden Laced Cochins and Barred Cochins, breeds originally from China (like all chickens), covered with parallel bars of alternating dark and light colors that shimmer like MC Escher paintings.

The Buff Orpingtons, a British breed, are the color of pure gold. The Silver Spangled Hamburgs sport greenish-black spangles on silvery-white plumage. The Rhode Island Reds and New Hampshire Reds, old-time favorites on American farms, are the color of bricks.

The Araucana hens, whose name comes from the Indian tribe in Chile where they were first discovered, have tufts of feathers growing from their ears like mutton-chops. (Yes, chickens have ears.) Araucana have become famous for laying "Easter" eggs in shades of blue and green.

At the large end of the scale, there's the Black Giant, an imposing breed developed in New Jersey that could be a bouncer for a bar in the same state. The Black Tailed Buff, a Japanese breed with golden plumage and a long black tail like a mocking bird, is among the most diminutive.

Quail Hill's rooster is a White Cochin, smaller than many of the hens, whose mellow demeanor is highly unusual for roosters, and may result from his formidable harem. He struts his head-to-toes downy plumage like a plush white Phat Farm leisure suit.

First prize for showiness goes to the Golden Polish, the Sir Elton John of the flock with its blue-iridescent legs and a "top hat" of feathers that it struts like a Las Vegas showgirl. (Some feathers missing from her top hat indicate that she's at the bottom of the pecking order.)

All the birds are rare breeds, which means they have fallen out of commercial favor, and their populations have reached perilously low levels. They are not suited for the standardized rigors of modern chicken farming, but they thrive under a range of other conditions. Think of them as a genetic insurance policy to ensure that we still have eggs regardless of what chicken diseases emerge or how our climate changes.

But it's the Jim Henson quality that largely explains why Quail Hill keeps the birds.

"I'm not sure which came first, the hen coop or the tire swing," says Scott Chaskey, officially known as the Preserve Manager but who prefers the title "farmer." "But they're built in the same place." When children visit the farm, they immediately flock to the coop.

The birds have multiple purposes like Quail Hill itself, set up by the Peconic Land Trust in 1990 as the nation's first community farm managed by a land trust. The farm includes 25 certified organic acres and serves 150 families. "The hens take dust baths, keep down aphids and weeds, and help prepare the soil for our winter greenhouse crops," says field manager Matt Celona.

And then there are the precious eggs ranging in color from the ordinary white and brown to the more unusual turquoise, deep olive and even pink. Farm members get a half-dozen eggs each week on a first-come-first-serve basis, but they consistently run out. (Other local sources of eggs and butchered chickens include North Sea Farms off Noyac Road in Southampton and Iacono Farms on Long Lane in East Hampton.)

Hens start laying around 18 to 20 weeks after they hatch and starting a flock is remarkably easy and inexpensive. Twenty-five female hatchlings will cost you between $35 and $50, depending on the breed. Murray McMurray in Webster City, Iowa, is the oldest rare breed hatchery in the United States and ships birds by airmail to arrive at your post office the following morning. They also sell ducks, turkeys, pheasants and other fowl, as well as feed, feeders, waterers, brooders, and paraphernalia like the Hom-Pik-Deluxe automatic feather picker, "the best backyard automatic picker you can buy."

—*Brian Halweil*

Dead Farmstands

Can you place these old farmstands?

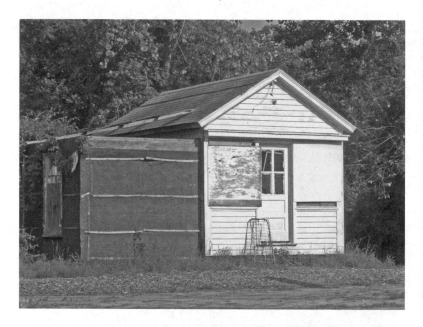

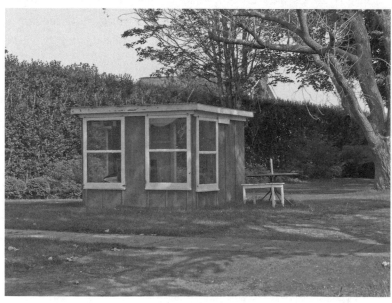

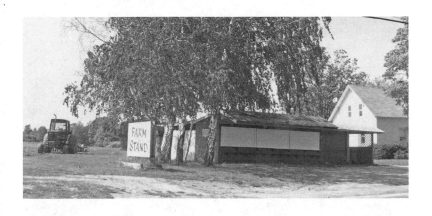

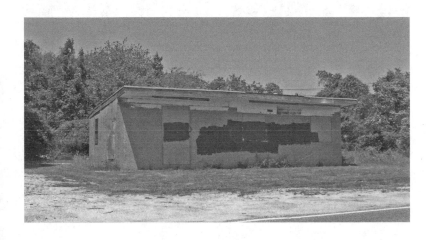

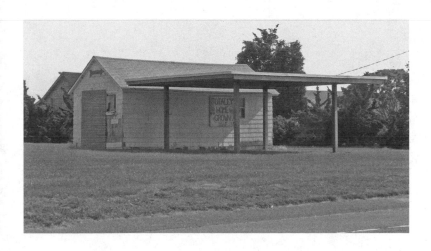

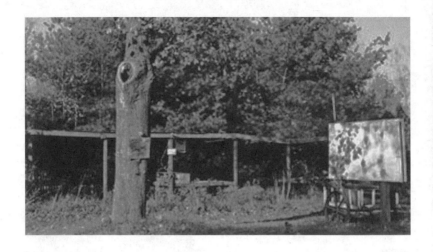

Long Island Growers' Markets

In 1998 Fred Terry, one of the numerous farmers in the New York area who participated in the New York City Greenmarket program, was approached by Islip resident Ellen Rossi about establishing a farmers market in her hometown. He immediately agreed. As the proprietor with his wife Ethel of a 130-acre farm in Orient Point in operation for almost 400 years he understood that the farmers market concept was one of key strategies for saving family farms.

He'd seen it work in New York City. When farmers sell into the wholesale market, not only do they have no control over the price of their produce, they give up most of the value to middlemen, truckers, and packagers. When they sell direct to consumers, — as they do in farmers markets — they keep 100% of the margin, and control prices. This gives them a chance to survive in the world of corporate agribusiness.

The Islip farmers markets was an immediate success. Suburbanites were just as eager as city folk to get their hands on fresh, local produce. Soon, other Long Island farmers were interested in participating, and other communities wanted their own local farmers markets.

In 2001 Fred's wife Ethel took over management of what was now a not-for-profit organization called Long Island Growers Markets. A dozen farms are now involved, serving nine local farmers markets on Long Island. LIGM has strict rules: you can sell only what you "make, bake, grow, or catch." And all participants are "hands-on": what they sell is what they pick. The personal relationship that develops between farmer and buyer is one of the rewards. Any producer enjoys and benefits from direct feedback from his customers.

There are other benefits, as well. all the farmers markets are situated at downtown sites, which brings traffic. Local merchants have started opening extra hours during the markets to serve that traffic.

The LIGM also participates in a couple of interesting federal programs. The WIC program issues once-a-year $24 vouchers for Women with Infants or small Children to be spent at farmers markets (only for fruits and vegetables, not baked goods or sweets.) After they've spent their vouchers, they usually come back, having discovered the pleasure (and economy) of buying fresh produce. Similarly a program for senior citizens offers an annual $18 voucher to be spent at farmers markets.

There are also three Long Island farmers markets not associated with the LIGM. The Sag Harbor market was founded in 2004, the Westhampton Beach market in 2005, and the East Hampton market in 2006.

Long Island Farmers Markets

New Hyde Park Farmers Market

Long Island Jewish Hospital
New Hyde Park, NY 11040
631-323-3653

Proprietor: Long Island Growers' Markets

Season: June 14 to Thanksgiving.

Hours: Wednesdays, 11 A.M. to 2 P.M.

Products: A wide variety of fruits, vegetables, plants, baked goods and more. All local products from at least ten local farms and purveyors.

About: The newest LIG market, started in 2006.

Hempstead Farmers Market

Christ First Presbyterian Church
Hempstead, NY 11549
631-323-3653

Proprietor: Long Island Growers' Markets

Directions: Located across from police department.

Season: July 7 to Thanksgiving.

Hours: Fridays, 7 A.M. to noon.

Products: A wide variety of fruits, vegetables, plants, baked goods and more. All local products from at least ten local farms and purveyors.

Locust Valley Farmers Market

Locust Valley, NY 11560

631-323-3653

Proprietor: Long Island Growers' Markets

Directions: Located across from police department.

Season: June 3 to Thanksgiving.

Hours: Saturdays, 8 A.M. to 1 P.M.

Products: A wide variety of fruits, vegetables, plants, baked goods and more. All local products from at least ten local farms and purveyors.

Lynbrook Farmers Market

Lynbrook, NY 11563

631-323-3653

Proprietor: Long Island Growers' Markets

Directions: Located at the railroad parking lot, corner of Sunrise Highway and Forest Ave.

Season: May 21 to Thanksgiving.

Hours: Sundays, 8 A.M. to 1 P.M.

Products: A wide variety of fruits, vegetables, plants, baked goods and more. All local products from at least ten local farms and purveyors.

Huntington Farmers Market

Elm Street
Huntington, NY 11743
631-323-3653

Proprietor: Long Island Growers' Markets

Directions: Located at Elm Street parking lot on Route 25A.

Season: May 21 to Thanksgiving.

Hours: Sundays, 8 A.M. to 1 P.M.

Products: A wide variety of fruits, vegetables, plants, baked goods and more. All local products from at least ten local farms and purveyors.

Islip Farmers Market

Montauk Highway
Islip, NY 11751
631-323-3653

Proprietor: Long Island Growers' Markets

Directions: Located at Town Hall parking lot on Montauk Hwy.

Season: May 20 to Thanksgiving.

Hours: Saturdays, 7 A.M. to noon.

Products: A wide variety of fruits, vegetables, plants, baked goods and more. All local products from at least ten local farms and purveyors.

About: Started in 1998, this was the first of the Long Island Growers' Markets.

Patchogue Farmers Market

Montauk Highway and Route 112
Patchogue, NY 11772
631-323-3653

Proprietor: Long Island Growers' Markets

Directions: Located at 7-Eleven parking lot on corner of Montauk Highway and Rte. 112.

Season: July 7 to Thanksgiving.

Hours: Fridays, 8 A.M. to 1 P.M.

Products: A wide variety of fruits, vegetables, plants, baked goods and more. All local products from at least ten local farms and purveyors.

Port Jefferson Farmers Market

Port Jefferson, NY 11777
631-323-3653

Proprietor: Long Island Growers' Markets

Directions: Located at town parking lot next to ferry.

Season: July 6 to Thanksgiving.

Hours: Thursdays, 11 A.M. to 4 P.M.

Products: A wide variety of fruits, vegetables, plants, baked goods and more. All local products from at least ten local farms and purveyors.

Riverhead Farmers Market

Main St.
Riverhead, NY 11901
631-323-3653

Proprietor: Long Island Growers' Markets

Directions: Located at village parking lot south of Main St. near Peconic Ave.

Season: July 6 to Thanksgiving.

Hours: Thursdays, 11 A.M. to 4 P.M.

Products: A wide variety of fruits, vegetables, plants, baked goods and more. All local products from at least ten local farms and purveyors.

Westhampton Beach Farmers Market

Mill Road
Westhampton Beach, NY 11977
631-288-1559
fax 631-288-7696
elsie.collins@verizon.net

Proprietor: Elsie Collins

Directions: Located at parking lot on Mill Road.

Season: May to November 11.

Hours: Saturdays, 9 A.M. to 1 P.M.

Products: 23 vendors, organic farmers, producers, Mecox Bay and Catapano cheeses.

Sag Harbor Farmers Market

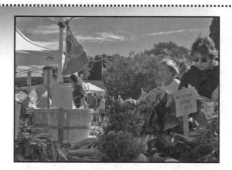

Bay St.
Sag Harbor, NY 11963
631-725-9133
*bhalweil@
worldwatch.org*

Proprietor: Kate Plumb

Directions: Located on east side of Marine Park on Bay St.

Season: June to November.

Hours: Saturdays, 9 A.M. to 1 P.M.

Products: Fruits, vegetables, cheeses, fish, plants, and more from local East End farms and purveyors.

About: The Sag Harbor Farmers Market was launched in September 2004, in conjunction with Harborfest, to provide residents with a source of fresh produce, to support local farmers and fishers, and to celebrate the agricultural history of the East End. The market runs every Saturday, from 9 to 1. It features twelve East End farmers and producers selling a wide range of produce, including organic vegetables, honey, cheese, clams and oysters, jams, and baked goods.

East Hampton Farmers Market

136 North Main St.
East Hampton, NY 11937

Directions: Parking lot of Nick & Toni's restaurant.

Season: July 5 to fall.

Hours: Wednesdays, 9 A.M. to 3 P.M.

For The Love Of Cheese

Mecox Bay Dairy
Mecox Road
Water Mill, NY

"I won't allow Art's Atlantic Mist in the house anymore." An inward smile of remembrance lit Stacy Ludlow's face. "I ate it morning, noon, and night..." the wife of the Bridgehampton cheesemaker sighed, "And gained 12 pounds." This side effect is unlikely to afflict anyone else, because Art Ludlow can't make enough of this ripe, runny, camembert-type cheese or his two other Mecox Bay Dairy cheeses to keep up with demand.

"Ludlow's cheese is unbelievable," says Charles Massoud, the urbane proprietor of Paumanok Vineyards, of the former potato farmer who went into the cheese-making business a mere year-and-a-half ago. "I think it's so good. It beats the European by a mile."

Atlantic Mist won "Best Product of the Year Award" from the East End Slow Food Convivium. Earlier, another of Ludlow's cheese, Mecox Sunrise, a firm, orange-skinned tomme-style cheese, won second place in its category at the American Cheese Competition in Milwaukee. At a recent Manhattan tasting of cheeses from 20 members of the New York State Farmstead Artisan Cheese Makers Guild, Atlantic Mist was a magnet for journalists and food professionals. It's not a shabby record for what 53-year-old Ludlow called his "test year" to see if cheese making was a viable business.

It also is no accident. Though a fledgling in cheese-making circles, Ludlow experimented from 1992 to 1998 making cheeses with milk from the lone family cow. Then he set about acquiring what in dairy circles are regarded as bovine Mercedes or Porsches – Jersey cows.

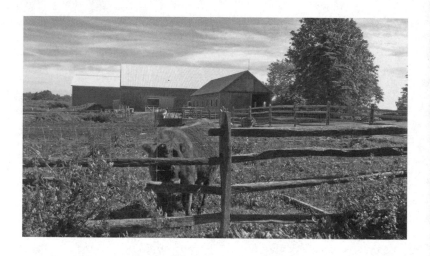

Actually, Ludlow had intended to market their milk as non-homogenized, creamline when he moved out of potatoes. "I bought a pasteurizer and got it all set up to go, and got a bottler." Both lie idle, never used, because orders for his cheeses outstrip the weekly 60 to 120 pounds of milk his cows contribute. It takes ten pounds of milk to make a pound of cheese, and each cow averages 30 pounds of milk a week.

Ludlow pondered the question: "Why do your cheeses taste so good?" First, he said the fat content of Jersey milk at 5 to 6% is off-the-charts compared to a more average top fat content of 4% from most cows, and it contains more solid protein as well. Both are important in quality cheese. "My sense is that flavor is pretty much dependent upon diet," he said. His current contingent of five adult cows and three young ones graze half the year on pastures that haven't been touched by chemicals for 30 years, and on hay and pelleted feed in the winter.

"The raw milk factor is a big one in flavor," he said, explaining that enzymes and proteins that develop flavor are destroyed even by low-temperature pasteurization. Aging raw-milk cheese over 60 days (as required by law) eliminates any harmful bacteria, but allows exceptional taste to emerge.

Add in the free-wheeling microbes of Mecox and you begin to develop the unique flavors of regional cheese that vary with the season and with what rides on the wind. Ludlow washes his wheels of Mecox Sunrise with water and salt. A revered bacteria in the cheese world which helps lend heft to Limburger and sensuousness to Epoisse – B. Linens or brevi bacteria linens – emerges spontaneously from the Bridgehampton air to coat Ludlow's cheese with an orange rind. "Opportunistic" East End molds fleck another pungent tomme-type, Shawondasse.

Ludlow hopes to breed his current Jersey crew into a "closed" herd of 20, without adding any outside animals with their potential for introducing disease. "My timetable is totally dependent on the girls in pasture."

As a sideline, Ludlow, who earned a B.S. from Cornell, has raised turkeys since high school and annually sells 250 on special order for Thanksgiving. Art and his brother Harry, who now raises vegetables for his Mecox Road farmstand, inherited the 100-acre Bridgehampton family farm on the death of their father over 35 years ago, then raised potatoes as their father and grandfather before them.

You'll find Ludlow's cheeses at Sag Harbor's Cavaniola Gourmet Cheese Shop priced at $18.99 a pound, and The Village Cheese Shop in Mattituck, at Westhampton Beach's Tierra Mar Restaurant and at Alison on School Street in Bridgehampton.

"I'm working harder than I did with potatoes, but I'm not looking back, and I'm enjoying it more," says Ludlow. So, one suspects, does Stacy.

—Geraldine Pluenneke

The Spirit of the Bees

Hamptons Honey Company
153 Little Noyac Path
Water Mill, NY

Mary Woltz recently had a once-in-a-lifetime experience. At least for a beekeeper.

"I saw two tooting and quacking queens," she said recently, standing over what looks like a chest of drawers sitting among rows of vegetables at the Green Thumb Organic Farm in Watermill.

In this rarely witnessed event, two queen bees — not one — hatch to replace the recently departed queen. "The secondary queen always toots, and the tertiary queen always quacks," Mary explained. She made the sounds of a train and a duck that she heard coming from the hive. The two queens can coexist for a little while, maintaining their own broods within the same hive. But sooner or later, in the battle for their tiny universe, one prevails.

Mary beamed, as if she were recounting a chance encounter with a movie star. She was almost as excited as Frédéric Rambaud, who listened intently and pouted, "I'm so jealous."

Beyond this interest in tooting and quacking queens — and an almost karmic connection to bees: both Frédéric and Mary "talk to the bee spirit" — the two share little in the way of background.

Frédéric grew up in urban Senegal and Paris. He worked in fashion and, later, in the mail-order gift business, where he had a knack for spotting the next big thing. This will be his first winter without concrete under his feet.

Mary grew up in rural North Carolina. Her eclectic past includes a stint as the wife of an Australian sheep rancher and as the general manager for Angelica's Kitchen in Manhattan.

But the two are now intimately linked by their common devotion to the honeybee and the latest local venture that revolves around the gracious pollinator: the Hamptons Honey Company.

"There is only one question to ask when beekeeping," Mary said. "What is best for the bees?" Standard beekeeping dogma would, in contrast, ask "What is most convenient for the bee-keeper?" "What is most efficient?" What will maximize honey production?" After all, raising bees and producing honey are not the same thing.

"Basically, the bee has become a factory farmed animal," Frédéric explained. Commercial beekeepers often feed the hives sugar-water so that more of the honey is available for harvest. They use pre-molded plastic honeycombs so that the bees don't waste energy building their combs. The industry uses cloned queens, and the more genetically uniform hives are plagued by parasitic mites, which beekeepers treat with antibiotics.

Bees on antibiotics?

Frédéric had a different vision. In 2001, he and his partner Alan Ceppos moved form New York City to Blue Spruce Farm, the 15-acre horse farm they purchased in Water Mill. What brought them out to the Hamptons? "Psychoanalysis," Frédéric joked. "For me, it was really a mid-life crisis. I wanted to do something more connected to my heart and my soul. I wanted to do something with nature."

His crash-course in this new lifestyle included training in nonagressive horsemanship ("a horse-whisperer sort of thing") and native plant species identification. He became a Citizen Pruner with Trees New York, and a Guerilla Gardener in organic horticulture.

His introduction to bees came during a nine-month course in biodynamic agriculture at the Pfeiffer Center in Chestnut Ridge, New York. Biodynamics, an approach to farming developed by Austrian philosopher Rudolf Steiner in the early 20th century, melds a sophisticated understanding of ecological processes with a faith in the power of the moon, sun, planets and other cosmic forces to influence crops. (More information is available at www.biodynamics.com.) In the case of bees, biodynamic practices include using wooden bee boxes, no plastic honeycombs, and herbal remedies for sick hives.

The idea behind this more gentle approach is that the bees are stronger and healthier over the long-term. "I consider my bees as my partners, and not as cheap labor," Frédéric said. "I talk to the bees just like I would talk to a pet."

"Or a friend," Mary corrected.

With his new skills, Frédéric searched for a venture that could use the property's woodlots, pasture, stables, and barn. (He still flirts with the idea of a retirement home for New York City Police Department horses.) When he heard that long-time local beekeeper Don Sausser was getting ready to retire, he jumped at the opportunity to purchase the business.

With 90 hives spread as far as East Moriches and Orient Point, Frédéric quickly realized that he would need someone to manage the hives as he developed the honey brand. That's when Mary entered the picture.

Frédéric first met Mary during his time at the Pfeiffer Center, where she was managing the garden and education programs, and was something of a prodigy. She had joined the Center to assist beekeeping guru Gunther Hauk. With no prior experience with bees — she holds a master's degree in landscape architecture — she displayed an uncanny understanding of the insects, a sort of inter-species kinship, and was quickly helping Hauk teach workshops. When Mary's tenure at the

Center ended, Frédéric invited her to the East End to be his master beekeeper.

During Mary's first weekend visit, Frédéric arranged a dinner with neighbors to give her a sense of the community. One more visit was enough. The rugged southern belle was sold — first, on the idea of managing an apiary, second, on the fact that it was in the cosmo-bucolic Hamptons.

The coupling was symbiotic. Her forte was in beekeeping, and his was in packaging, labels, design, and marketing.

On a crisp, sunny day in late September, the two worked side-by-side, collecting the last honey of the season. The harsh winter and cold, damp spring meant slim pickings. "We lost 20 percent of our hive last winter," Frédéric said. "We had the labels ready for strawberry and black locust honey, but the blossoms were rained off."

Mary wore clogs, long pants, a sleeveless top, and an orange bandana that holds back her hair. A veil and other standard beekeeper paraphernalia make it harder to "listen to the bees' mood," she said. (For stings, she searches the ground for plantain, a common weed with anti-inflammatory properties, tears off a few leaves and chews them into an easy-to-apply poultice.)

"I just have to laugh when I open a hive, because it's filled with joy," Mary said, chuckling and puffing a bit of herb-infused smoke at the humming stack of boxes. "Bees are sun-beings. They hate the rain. They live to work."

"Mary's a bee-girl," Frédéric added, as if he was teasing her about a school-girl crush.

Or, to put it another way. "When the bees sting Mary, she says 'Thank you,'" Frédéric quipped as he put on a veil. "When they sting me, I say something that's not printable."

Just as modern beekeeping has become sterile and automated, Frédéric hopes to take the industrialization out of honey eating. Most store-bought honey has been heated to 200 degrees Fahrenheit to prevent crystallization during long shelf-lives and "so you can easily squeeze it out of your teddy bear," Frédéric noted. The heating destroys enzymes and certain nutrients, not to mention what it does to subtle aromas and flavors. All of Frédéric's honey is raw and unfiltered, jarred in a room connected to his horsestable.

And instead of the generic blends of honey from various locales and seasons, Frédéric envisions vintages specific to the plant cycles of the East End. Black locust honey. Apple, blueberry, and strawberry blossom honey. Even zucchini blossom honey.

"This is about provenance, local cuisine, Slow Food," Frédéric said. "About educating the palate." He developed the new Hamptons Honey brand for the varietal blends, while maintaining the well-known Don Sausser label for wildflower and clover honeys. The honeys are sold at local farmstands and stores, used in Jessie's brand of baked goods, and served in the five-star Ross School cafeteria.

But it's not just about honey. Frédéric and Mary envision a nonprofit research center that will refine "an organic approach" to beekeeping (They keep meticulous records.), and offer classes for hobbyists and entrepreneurs. "The nonprofit will create bee yards and bee habitat throughout the Hamptons," Frédéric said. He is converting his own property to a bee sanctuary by pulling out invasive plants and seeding a meadow of native wildflowers.

In this sense, the venture is part of building a healthy landscape. The bees help pollinate crops, and the farmers help create a bee-friendly landscape. (Frédéric and Mary favor sites on organic farms, since exposure to pesticides is one of the reasons for the sharp decline in the nation's bee populations.) Frédéric and Mary are also contacting large landowners to use part of their land for "bee fodder."

"Our sites are really the best of the Hamptons landscape," Frédéric said. The margins of meadows. The middles of farm fields and orchards. Frédéric described one Sagaponack site where he can see and smell the ocean while he tends the hives. He looked to the horizon and guessed, "It's probably the most expensive bee field in the world."

—*Brian Halweil*

Community Supported Agriculture

One of the newest trends in farming is CSA — Community Supported Agriculture. Families and individuals subscribe to a season's worth of produce and pick up their bounty weekly. Farmers benefit because they have a guaranteed level of income and can set prices that cover costs. Buyers benefit from an ever-changing stream of farm-fresh produce and save time shopping.

CSAs are extremely popular. As we went to press in June, nearly all Long Island CSA subscriptions had been sold out for the 2006 season. Make a note to call early next year.

Some CSAs require subscribers to put in a certain number of hours per week, some don't. (Go for the ones that do: you need the exercise!)

The Golden Earthworm farm is the most active CSA farmer on Long Island but Garden of Eve, HOG, and Sophia Garden are oversubscribed, too. On the East End The Green Thumb was a pioneer, and Quail Hill and Sang Lee offer CSA subscriptions at their farms.

EECO Farm in East Hampton takes the concept one step further offering private garden plots to more than 100 subscribers. Expect this community garden trend to take off next.

Golden Earthworm CSA:

Holbrook
125 Tremper Street
Holbrook, NY 11741
TUESDAY pickup 12–8

Huntington
2 Bouton Place
Huntington, NY 11743
TUESDAY pickup 2:30–8

Jamesport (farm)
652 Peconic Bay Blvd.
Jamesport, NY 11947
WEDNESDAY pickup 11–8

Massapequa Park
91 Laurel Drive
Massapequa Park, NY 11762
TUESDAY pickup 3:15 -8

Port Jefferson
1 Chips Court
Port Jefferson, NY 11777
TUESDAY pickup 1–8

Port Washington
Om Sweet Om Yoga
37 Avenue A
Port Washington, NY 11050
Home delivery also available.
THURSDAY pickup 3–4. Friday from 9–11

Ridge
5 Niewood Drive
Ridge, NY 11961
TUESDAY pickup 11–8

Rockville Centre
66 S. Lewis Place
Rockville Centre, NY 11570
TUESDAY pickup 3:30–8

Sea Cliff
Roots Restaurant

242 Sea Cliff Avenue
Sea Cliff, NY 11579
THURSDAY pickup 2–TBD.

Smithtown
41 Brooksite Drive
Smithtown, NY 11787
TUESDAY pickup 1:30 -8

St. James
23 Ashleigh Drive
St. James, NY 11780
TUESDAY pickup 1:30–8

Stony Brook
124 Christian Avenue
Stony Brook, NY 11790
TUESDAY pickup 1:30–8

Stony Brook University
Stony Brook Union Loading Dock
Stony Brook University Campus
Local Contact: Lisa Ospitale, 631-632-6529
THURSDAY pickup 12–4. Friday 8:30–12. Please bring ID.

Valley Stream
96 Foster Avenue
Valley Stream, NY 11580
TUESDAY pickup 3:30–8

If you are interested in joining the CSA through any of the following groups, please contact them directly. Thank you.

Douglaston, Queens
718-229-4000 ext. 212
Alley Pond Environmental Center
22806 Northern Blvd.
Douglaston, NY

Forest Hills, Queens
Dennis Redmond
718-592-5757 Ext. 286
foresthillscsa@yahoo.com

Jackson Heights, Queens
pickup at St. Mark's Church
Corner of 82nd and 34th Avenue
Jackson Heights, NY
718-512-5097

Garden of Eve CSA:

Manhasset
Pick up for this CSA is at the Reconstructionist Synagogue of
the North Shore located on Plandome Road in Manhasset, on
Wednesdays from approximately 4–7.

Riverhead
At the farmstand

Also Brooklyn and Upper West Side Manhattan.

Hamlet Organic Garden CSA:

Bayshore
425 Pine Ave
Bayshore, NY
Contact persons: Rich and Lisa Richards, 631-206-3047
WEDNESDAY pickup 3:30-6:30

Setauket
15 Balin Avenue
South Setauket, NY

Contact person: Stephanie Regan 631-648-8354
WEDNESDAY pickup 3:30-6:30

Sophia Garden CSA:

555 Albany Avenue
Amityville, NY 11707
631-842-6000 x 307

The Green Thumb CSA:

Water Mill and Huntington.

Quail Hill Community Farm CSA:

At the farm in Amagansett.

Sang Lee CSA:

At the farm in Peconic.

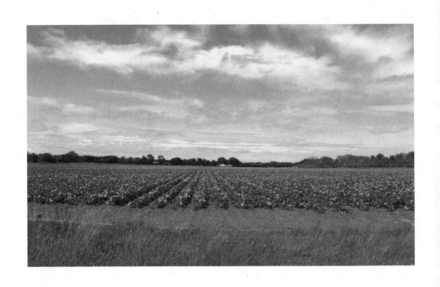

Long Island Farm Bureau

The Farm Bureau is a wonderful and unique American concept.

Farm Bureaus are true grassroots, member-driven organizations with a century's legacy in political activism. Farm bureaus are private, non-partisan, not-for-profit agricultural membership and advocacy organizations known as "The Voice of Commercial Agriculture." In Nassau and Suffolk counties the Long Island Farm Bureau is the Voice of Long Island Agriculture.

The mission of LIFB is to fairly and aggressively represent and serve the best interests of their members through united action, using the strength of a grassroots organizational structure and relying on effective leadership to provide strong, networked and allied Farm Bureau organizations at the local, state, and national organization levels. The collective goal: to protect and strengthen the nation's agricultural industry.

That especially includes the agricultural industries of the Long Island region and of New York State, where Suffolk County is the state's largest dollar producer of agricultural products.

- LIFB members employ more than 8,000 people in the Long Island region.

- Member production areas are near to both wholesale and retail markets.

- Suffolk County #1 in Market Value of products in New York State.

- $168 million in value of agricultural products.

- More than 400 farms in Suffolk County, with 33,000+ acres in use.

- Four farms remain active in Nassau County.

- $1 billion total economic impact for regional economy.

- More than 100 different crops grown on Long Island.

For more information:

631-727-3777
AskUs@lifb.com
lifb.com

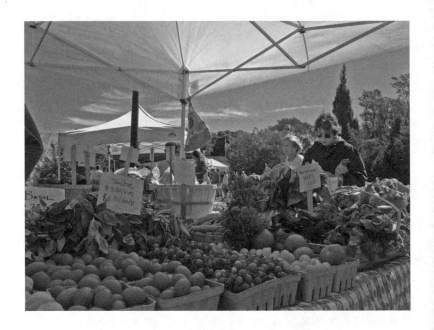

Slow Food USA

The East End Convivium of Slow Food USA was founded in October 2003 by Ted Conklin, proprietor of the famed American Hotel in Sag Harbor, together with Mary Foster Morgan, Tom Morgan, Kate Plumb, and writer Brian Halweil.

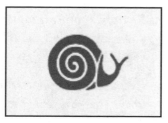

It was an immediate success, hosting dinners that focused on local produce, seafood, wine and beer at many of the area's most interesting restaurants, including the American Hotel, Star Boggs, Nick & Toni's, the Ram's Head Inn, and Tierra Mar.

Legend has it that the Slow Food movement began in Italy 20 years ago when the first McDonald's opened in Rome. and a group protested by getting together to eat real food.

The founding father of the Slow Food Movement, Carlo Petrini, recognized in 1986 that the industrialization of food was standardizing taste and leading to the annihilation of thousands of food varieties and flavors. Concerned that the world was quickly reaching a point of no return, he wanted to reach out to consumers and demonstrate to them that they have choices over fast food and supermarket homogenization. He rallied his friends and began to speak out at every available opportunity. Soon the movement was born and Slow Food was created. Today the organization is active in 50 countries and has a worldwide membership of over 80,000.

The East End Convivium has the following goals:

1. Educational events and public outreach that encourage the enjoyment of pure foods that are local, seasonal, and organically grown.

2. Caring for the land of the East End and protecting the biodiversity of our community for the benefit of future generations.

3. Identification, promotion, and protection of economically and ecologically fragile East End animals, plants, fruits, and vegetables.

4. Respect and support for East End artisans who grow, produce, market, and prepare wholesome foods, wines, and spirits.

5. The revival of the kitchen and the table as centers of pleasure, culture and economy.

6. Promoting a slower, more harmonious rhythm of life.

For more information:
  slowfoodlongisland.org
  slowfoodusa.org
  slowfood.com

  Mary@edibleeastend.com
  tbc3@theamericanhotel.com

Edible East End

Founded in 2005 by editor Brian Halweil and publisher Stephen Munshin, *Edible East End* is a quarterly magazine that celebrates the harvest of the Hamptons and North Fork. Filled with stories and photography, *Edible East End* is helping to define Long Island cuisine, promote the local bounty, and build ties between farmers, fishers, and the rest of the community. By demonstrating just how

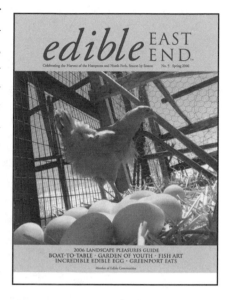

much our landscape offers, the magazine and website point readers towards the region's wine, seafood, produce, food shops and restaurants.

According to the publishers eating local isn't just good for our health, farmers, and the planet. It's also a growing nationwide trend. *Edible East End* is part of Edible Communities, a network of more than two dozen local food publications from coast to coast.

Everywhere you look there are signs that the East End is in the midst of a culinary renaissance. *Edible* wants to spread the word.

For more information:
  POB 779
  Sag Harbor 11963
  Phone: 631 537 4637
  info@edibleeastend.com
  edibleeastend.com

Web References

More information about Eastern Long Island:
  Peconic.org

Slow Food USA:
  Slowfood.com, SlowFoodUSA.org

Slow Food East End Convivium:
  SlowfoodLongIsland.org

Edible East End magazine:
  Edibleeastend.com

Sustainable seafood:
  Montereybayaquarium.org/cr/seafoodwatch.asp

Organic Consumers Association:
  Organicconsumers.org

The national local farm scene:
  Localharvest.org

The Long Island Farm Bureau:
  LIFB.com

New York Farms organization:
  NYFarms.info

Northeast Organic Farmers Association, New York chapter:
  NOFANY.org

New York State Natural Heritage Program:
  NYNHP.org

Union of Concerned Scientists Food project:
  www.ucsusa.org/food_and_environment/

Guide to East End Resources:
  EastEndCommunity.com

Stony Brook Center for Wine, Food, and Culture:
  stonybrook.edu/winecenter/

The Stony Brook University Center for Wine, Food, and Culture was founded in 2004 for the purpose of bringing together people and ideas that convey and sustain cultural connections to food and wine.

About the Contributors

Robbi Goldberg, who graciously provided the paintings that you see on the cover, is a self-taught painter with an MBA in international business from George Washington University. From 1983 to 1996 she lived and painted full time on the Greek island of Ios. Her aim was to produce a record of a vanishing way of life. This work was widely shown throughout Greece, and in Berlin, Israel, Moscow, and Washington DC.

For several years now Robbi has been working on a series of acrylic on canvas paintings of East End farmstands. from which the "postcards" on our cover were derived. These paintings were offered in a successful show at the Castello di Borghese winery gallery in 2005-2006.

Giclée prints of these paintings are available for purchase. Please visit *Peconic.org* for more information.

Brian Halweil is a writer and editor specializing in food and farming issues. He was one of the founders of the East End Convivium of Slow Food, active in establishing the Sag Harbor Farmers Market, and a founder of *Edible East End*, where he serves as editor. Brian is also the author of *Eat Here: Homegrown Pleasures in a Global Supermarket* (New York: Norton, 2004), a fascinating book that should be essential reading for anyone interested in real food.

Geraldine Pluenneke is a writer and reporter of wide experience currently working on a book based on interviews with 160 top chefs across Europe and America on why food from industrial agriculture has lost its flavor, and how to shop and cook to get flavor back. Her stories appear often in *Newsday, Dan's Papers* and elsewhere. She lives in Montauk. "To me, the wonderful flavors and extra nutrients of just- picked local produce, are more than enough reason for anyone to drive extra miles to shop at farmstands."

Send Us More Info

This is the first edition of the *HEP Guide to Long Island Farmstands*. Undoubtedly we've missed one or more of your favorites. Let us know! Email *Jim@Peconic.org* with your comments and suggestions. Your reviews of the farmstands and farmers markets where you shop are also welcome.

Thank you!